BE
YOUR OWN
DOCTOR

BE
YOUR OWN
DOCTOR

Let LIVING FOOD
Be Your Medicine

ANN WIGMORE

AVERY PUBLISHING GROUP
Wayne, New Jersey

The medical and health procedures in this book are based on the training, personal experiences, and research of the author. Because each person and situation is unique, the author and publisher urge the reader to check with a qualified health professional before using any procedure where there is any question as to its appropriateness.

The publisher does not advocate the use of any particular diet and exercise program, but believes the information presented in this book should be available to the public.

Because there is always some risk involved, the author and publisher are not responsible for any adverse effects or consequences resulting from the use of any of the suggestions, preparations, or procedures in this book. Please do not use the book if you are unwilling to assume the risk. Feel free to consult a physician or other qualified health professional. It is a sign of wisdom, not cowardice, to seek a second or third opinion.

CONTENTS

PREFACE

Twenty-five years ago, I established the Hippocrates Health Institute (now world wide in scope) in order to develop my ideas on sprouting seeds and growing indoor greens. Through long and careful observation of myself and others, I found that when we give our bodies the rich nourishment they need from living foods, and when we work in close harmony with Nature's laws, Nature's boundless healing power will always be there to assist us.

I also observed the endless problems resulting from our neglect of these laws. Such neglect can have a devastating effect on us all.

My own personal struggles with colitis, headaches, arthritis, and a host of other problems led me to change my lifestyle. I changed my diet and my mental attitudes; I began to exercise. A new pattern of life unfolded for me and prepared me for sharing and teaching my ideas, and then I realized that I was meant to be healthy and productive and to live a long life.

I became convinced that although our times are troubled and dangerous, they also offer us a great opportunity, for we can change ourselves and our course of events by teaching others about Nature's laws. One of the best ways to do this is to open their eyes to living foods, for the key to longevity and health, as I have found for myself, is enzyme nourishment through living foods, regular exercise, and a happy and healthy attitude.

On such a strong foundation we can build healthy bodies and live longer, richer lives, and by bringing healthy children into the world we can participate in our role as co-creator with God. Will you join me in my desire for one peaceful world? Such a world is possible if each one of us will turn to nature for living nourishment and for an understanding of our purpose in life.

Ann Wigmore, 1982

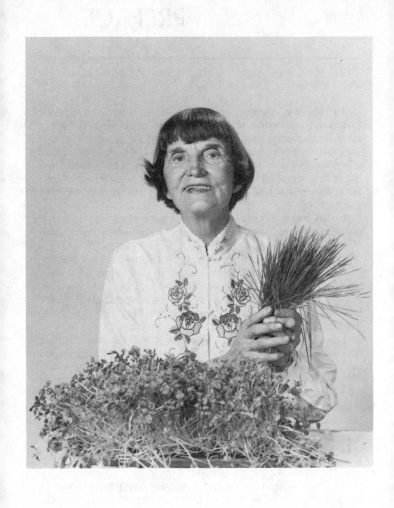

Ann Wigmore, founder of the Hippocrates Health Institute.

Part I

The Road to Health

INTRODUCTION

Disease stems from deficiencies and a lack of understanding of Mother Nature's laws of health, plus the unwillingness to accept the obligation to keep the precious temple—the body —in order. This is accomplished by keeping it clean and well-nourished. And, of course, providing necessary aids such as rest, relaxation, positive thinking and plenty of exercise through hard work.

How unfortunate it is that we have become dependent upon others to take care of our mental, physical and spiritual duties. When our spiritual leader explains HIS spiritual beliefs, we gulp them down as gospel. When the psychologist explains the methods our thinking should be geared to, we accept the instructions without questioning. When the physician tells us to take this and that, we accept the suggestions as ultimatums. And when we find ourselves in predicaments, we usually blame others for our difficulties.

We fail to learn how to think for ourselves and to take care of our bodies properly by asking for the guidance which is always there for us to utilize instantly and which will amply provide for our individual needs. Our bodies definitely let us know whether or not we are treating them right or wrong. When we are well, we feel relaxed and happy and energy is unlimited. When we are ill, we have pains, uneasiness and our minds are filled with fear. We must understand the warnings which are given us—and heed them. This will help us maintain and regain the health which is our birthright.

Since most health problems result from deficiencies, the vital need is nourishment and that nourishment has to be unprocessed and uncooked, and in addition grown in organic, earth. The reason the book *BE YOUR OWN DOCTOR, NATURE'S WAY* has come into being is the condition of the country. The following letters should convince you of the necessity for health education Mother Nature's way, as it places great emphasis on prevention of illness as well as healing and the elimination of health problems generally.

The heartbroken mother of an eighteen-year-old boy writes, "My reasons for ordering your books are—I have a handicapped son. He has been ill for four years. He first had surgery on the lower back, on the three lower vertebrae of the spine, because we were told they were defective. While recuperating from this operation, he started having a numbness of his left hand and foot. All the neurological tests were performed and the doctors, thinking there was a swelling of the brain, performed an exploratory operation, but nothing wrong was brought to light. Because of the first operation, a vertebra slipped out of place in his neck and had to be replaced through surgery. Then the real trouble started and now he can hardly walk, is partly paralyzed on his left side, and has double vision all the time.

"I had to turn to someone else because the medical doctors admitted they could do nothing more to help. I started him on vitamins and he is also taking twelve tissue salts as prescribed by a homeopathic doctor. Still my son has not improved any as far as health is concerned. I would like to bring him to your place because my husband passed on last November from a heart attack and too much surgery. Please help me to get my son back to health."

Such communications which have come to me during the past few years reveal a condition of ill health in this country that proves conclusively that there is little time left for theories —we must go back to fundamentals and each person must learn how to be his or her own doctor. It should be remembered that it is never to late to work with Mother Nature, that she never fails to help when she is provided with the proper tools. Any illness in one part of the body, including the spine, indicates a general deficiency in the body as a whole, manifesting in that weak spot. If the body had cooperated with Mother Nature, his back would have automatically healed itself. Fortunately, the young body generally responds quickly to the utilization of simple, natural methods.

Another letter from a distressed human being clearly indicates a household where nutritional deficiencies are marked. And, of course, there is probably the habit of eating too often and too much and wrong combinations. "I just came out of the hospital and have made the discouraging discovery that the complaint which took me into the hospital is worse than ever. I am a diabetic and now take large doses of insulin which has affected my eyesight adversely. I cannot read, even with glasses. To add to my troubles, when I got home I found out that my little granddaughter, nine years old, who is very thin, has worms and is anemic. Also, my little grandson, who is seven, has sinus trouble and my other granddaughter is a victim of sore throats, headaches and ear problems. Please help us."

Millions of dollars spent on "medical research", drugs and operations will not correct such conditions. This money would be more wisely spent teaching each person to understand the workings of their own human mechanism and how to keep their body in first-class running order. This household is only a sample of what is happening all through this country. Here is a letter from India from a distressed father whose two-month-old infant is suffering from a rare skin disease, epidermolysis; his other daughter, three years old, is also covered with sores and is considered incurable. "On the suggestion of a friend, I started to use the wheatgrass on my daughters and it immediately showed beneficial results. It is the best 'medicine' for them I have ever found. I wish to go into this matter more thoroughly now that I have seen the wondrous results which have helped so much the freeing of their misery."

The faulty diet of these parents, especially of a mother during pregnancy, caused the affliction of these children. I am sure that when this father adopts the living food program for the family, real progress in health will be made for the entire household. The reason he has these problems is because of

3

improper eating. The sufferer must remove the cause before Mother Nature can do her job and he can be healed. This is no CURE for anything. The body's health must be rebuilt before the body can heal itself. And to rebuild the body's health, we must feed the body living, organically grown, uncooked foods, Nature's way to health.

PRESENT DAY HEALTH

NEWSPAPER STATISTICS—*the State of Health in America*

"Forty-eight million people in the U.S.A. suffer from heart disease, and this, together with strokes, accounts for more than half the deaths in the United States each year."

"Twelve million people suffer from arthritic disease and ten million are burdened with neurological disorders."

"Four out of five persons 64 and over have disabilities or chronic disease."

"At least two million children are mentally retarded and 4 million are mentally disturbed."

"The National Association for Mental Health estimates that one out of every ten Americans—19 million in all—suffer from some sort of mental illness."

According to government statistics, some 67% of American school children under eleven years of age failed to pass the minimum physical fitness test, compared to but 9 per cent of European children in the same group.

We have the highest medical bills in the world. Our hospitals and doctors are overtaxed with labor. There is a need for a new approach. Dr. Spies has stated simply at the AMA annual convention in 1957, "If only we knew enough all diseases could be prevented and could be cured through proper nutrition."

Many folks do not care to admit they are sick or that natural health is on the downgrade. Nor do they think it necessary to use preventive measures. I would like you to check the following list and see just how you measure up. No person rates sound health if he does not answer the following satisfactorily:

Do you have a tobacco habit?
Do you use alcohol?
Are you utilizing painkillers or digestive aids?
Do you drink coffee or tea?
Are you free from nervous instability?
Are you always hungry and tend to overeat often?
Do you crave certain nourishment that you know is not suitable for you?
Are you happy and do you live a satisfying life?
Do you have sufficient faith to carry you through emergencies?
Are you generous?
Are you free from body odors including halitosis?
Do you have dental defects?
Has your hair turned grey and are there bald spots?
Do you have facial wrinkles and are you worried about aging?
Do you have adequate bowel movements? As many movements as you have meals each day?

Constipation is the greatest single menace, greatest health destroyer. If you do not meet these minimal health standards, you are either sick now or soon will be ailing. If you follow our suggested preventive program you will not only save time and expense but prevent overshadowing fear and degeneration.

Dr. Redding discovered malnutrition to cause much insanity. There are thousands of inmates of insane asylums as a result of starvation on full stomachs. Many children fail in their marks at school because their bodies lack the proper sustaining elements to feed their brain cells.

Invading germs seek some type of rubbish heap—toxinladen cells—where the environment is satisfactory for their growth. A wise doctor once said, "The only sickness which exists in the body is toxicity. Healthy cells, nourished properly, are immune to such attacks."

Through my work with sufferers with degenerated bodies, many have been completely renewed through the use of living, organically grown uncooked food.

An outstanding example of what proper nourishment can accomplish is shown in the case of a 93-year-old man. He had suffered a "stroke" the year before, heart trouble had affected his movements, and he underwent lapses of memory. Receiving proper living nourishment, organically grown, uncooked food, this individual restored his health to a state where he was more alert, vigorous and energetic than when he was fifty years old.

We had a visitor from Australia not long ago. She was very upset because she had aged so much in the past year. She was shocked when she looked at the passport picture taken of her but a year before. She was a spiritual leader who believed in the Almighty's help and yet her prayers were unanswered. I asked her about her health and she replied that she felt wonderful—yet she could not even lift her own traveling bag. She claimed a heart problem prevented her from doing so.

CANCER —

In the past ten years, the National Cancer Institute has spent over $7 billion on the war against cancer—almost three times as much as the federal agency's total funding during the previous 35 years of its existence. Last year an annual campaign of the American Cancer Society raised $150 million from Americans who believe that the only way to fight cancer is with a "check-up and a check." In 1979, for the first time in history, federal spending on cancer exceeded $1 billion in the U.S.A. That same year, 70,000 more Americans died of cancer than in 1971. In spite of the millions—in dollars as well as in lives—that have been sacrificed in the war against cancer, the conventional medical establishment cannot report an overall victory that might make these past losses worthwhile. Summing up the situation recently, two-time Nobel Prize winner Linus Pauling, Ph.D., wrote, "Everyone should know that the war on cancer is largely a fraud, and that the National Cancer Institute and American Cancer Society are derelict in their duties to the American people who support them."

In 1945, one out of fifteen died of cancer. When the war on cancer was first declared by the Nixon Administration in 1971, one in every six American deaths was due to the disease. By 1978, after billions had been spent on research of conventional methods of therapy, the rate was up to one in every five Americans. Current estimates are that cancer will cause one in every four deaths by 1988, one in every three by 2008, and one in two by the year 2025—a gloomy death sentence for those born today. Over the years, cancer will strike in approximately two out of three families. In the 1970s, there were an estimated 3.5 million deaths due to cancer, and more than 10 million people under medical care for cancer. In 1981, approximately 800,000 people were diagnosed as having cancer; another estimated 420,000 will die of the disease—1,150 a day, about one every 75 seconds.

Nearly a century of extensive research of conventional modes of treatment, including surgery, radiation, hormone therapy, immunotherapy, and chemotherapy, has produced no significant difference in overall cancer survival rates since 1950.

Scientists learned that diets high in fat and protein exerted a major influence on the origin and course of cancer. That cancer could be diet-related (and therefore diet-healed) is to me an exciting breakthrough. However, these encouraging findings were covered up and never applied because, in the words of NCI founder Dean Burke, Ph.D., "After World War II along came chemotherapy, which represented a more profitable and fashionable area of investigation."

In my work at the Hippocrates Health Institute, I have utilized the discoveries of science for over thirty years. We know that no known disease can penetrate the strength of a healthy body. A low protein, low starch, low fat and high enzyme, high vitamin, highly alkaline and high mineral diet is the key. Anyone can restore health by way of detoxification and rebuilding healthy cells so that the body can heal itself. Sickness is only a failure to understand the balance of the body, mind, and spirit, which creates well-being.

The Hippocrates regime consists of a diet of live fruits, vegetables, sprouts, and greens, as well as indoor planting, exercise, detoxification, education about the body's self-healing power, and a positive attitude.

My work has proven beyond a shadow of a doubt that

a healthy diet and a clean colon are most important in maintaining well-being. Constipation is the greatest crime against health, and a possible cause of cancer in many instances. From my observations, every indication points out that the healing power for overcoming cancer and other serious ailments is centered in our own kitchens and the food we grow and eat. Remember what Hippocrates said thousands of years ago: "Let food be thy medicine." The body's ability to get healthy and heal itself is evident, and no disease can exist when the bloodstream is clean and the cells are well nourished. Greens and sprouts will help keep the blood clean and the cells well nourished. When the cells are nourished, the circulation system is able to carry away wastes and toxins, thereby improving the health of the body. We have a wonderful cleaning system: the lungs, liver, kidneys, skin, and colon. We only need to learn about it so that we may cooperate with these vital helpers by nourishing them, keeping them clean, and allowing them to heal us.

Charles R. Shaw, M.D., University of Texas Cancer Center, recently found that sprouts can help protect us from cancer. In the experiment, his researchers exposed healthy bacteria to a cancer causing substance in the presence of an extract (juice) made from wheat sprouts. The cancer was inhibited up to ninety-nine percent using the sprout extract. Mung bean and lentil sprouts showed the same ability.

What to do. The best method in dealing with cancer problems is first to remove the cause. A diet containing uncooked nourishment will help to cleanse and rebuild the cells into a healthy state. Sprout juices with greens, wheatgrass juice, plenty of Rejuvelac and watermelon juice are all excellent.

Dr. Earp-Thomas, from long experience, fully convinced me that when cooked food is eaten, it permits tumors and cancer growths to build within the body. Yet when living food is substituted, the cancer and other growths immediately begin to shrink for lack of nourishment. The most thrilling experience I can recall was seeing cancer cells taken from a human body thriving on cooked food, but unable to survive on the same kind of food when it was uncooked. Such an experience taught me something that textbooks and teachers never can erase from my mind. For the human body, an uncooked vegetarian diet is the *only* type of nutrition. Cooked food is dead, and actually unsuitable as nourishment for the digestive processes of all animals, including human beings.

The role of nutrition in cancer has been confirmed by new scientific observations which recognize the fact that blood is often lacking in organic mineral elements, vitamins, enzymes: health-giving nutrients for creating vibrant cells. Cooked foods saturate the blood with waste and foreign matter, and as a safety measure, the body builds the cancerous cells from the blood pollutants at a rapid pace, reducing the impurities in the blood. On the other hand, during therapy the growths of cancer are brought piecemeal into the bloodstream, and removed through the eliminative organs. The anti-cancer diet consists of wheatgrass chlorophyll, juices from greens and sprouts, fruits, vegetables, seeds, and fermented foods, all eaten uncooked.

Terry Fox, one of many talented and gifted contributors to mankind, was afflicted with and died of cancer. John Wayne, the great movie star, died of lung cancer. Hubert H. Humphrey, one of the greatest political figures in the history of the United States, died of cancer of the colon. Ella Grasso, the Governor of Connecticut and the first woman ever elected governor in her own right, succumbed to liver cancer. It is unforgettable that these great contributors to the service of mankind should die prematurely at the peak of their careers. Living Foods are the key.

Fear of cancer comes from gossip, suggestions imbedded by the cancer drives and cancer safeguards that are reiterated everywhere in the press, by physicians, and in general conversation. These ideas settle dismally in the consciousness and often bring on the very thing we seek to avoid. By the same token, continuous thoughts of good health and how you can, through common sense, take adequate steps to eliminate cancerous conditions bring relief in ways that may seem miraculous.

HEART DISEASE —

Heart disease is still on the increase and remains one of the greatest sources of death in this country, especially among young men.

Dr. Paul Dudley White of Boston, once the world's leading heart specialist, is a leading advocate of dietary prevention to heart attacks. In Dr. White's opinion, undernutrition is not the most serious condition facing the public. Rather, it is that too much food is consumed by the average person and the multitude of calories in food is cause for alarm. After much careful study, nutritionists declare that one of the main causes of heart problems is the consumption of too much cholesterol taken into the body by animal fat. The experience of vegetarians proves this absolutely. Experiments reveal that the fatty content of meat lines the interior of the arteries, blocking the free flow of blood which places undue strain upon the heart often with fatal results.

The Bantu people of South Africa are famous among nutritionists for their freedom from coronary heart disease. The Bantu diet consists of less than 20% fat calories versus the American 40% plus. The existing implication of a rich animal fat diet as an important factor in the etiology of thrombosis is very strong. The countries which suffer the highest mortality from arteriosclerotic and degenerative heart disease include the U.S.A., New Zealand, Australia, Finland, Canada and the United Kingdom, where relatively large amounts of proteins with a high content of cyanocobolamin, and/or large quantities of pasturized milk products, are consumed.

There was a time when people worked hard for their food and they did not have the health problems that people have today who do not exert themselves. The modern individual sits in front of the television set with his hot dogs, cokes and tobacco. If he tends to die suddenly from heart trouble, it does not mean that the heart was the original cause. It indicates that he was already sick, that the trouble was clogged arteries and that the waste material in those arteries prevented the free flow of blood. Exercise helps to prevent the accumulation of this waste. Poorer individuals lacking too much food do not have this kind of arterial disease. An excessive amount of food in the stomach overworks the digestive organs.

A typical executive, in these modern times, may pass out after partaking of a large meal. The heart is not primarily at fault. The true cause of collapse is intestinal gas which prevents even circulation of the blood. The heart itself is generally uninvolved—at least, not directly. When the blood ceases to flow freely, the heart automatically stops beating. The situation is that simple. Yet millions of dollars are spent yearly in the vain hope of finding the "real cause".

This is Dr. Paul Dudley White's analysis of the conditions which cause the death of so many of our leaders. "A good executive is a human being who gets things done despite hardship, long hours, and the wear and tear upon the mentality. It is a sobering fact that if the executive is not a perfectionist, is content with doing his job complacently and without worry, such executive has a much better chance for survival than one who works, worries and indulges in too much food, too little exercise, and tobacco. An executive who is always under a great strain is a candidate for nervous prostration. Too much worry and nervous exhaustion are kin."

"Unfortunately," Dr. White continues, "the general excuse for the sudden termination of life is that the stress and strain of modern civilization is too great." At a recent psychiatric convention it was determined that the word "stress" merely meant "life". In fact, a human being cannot live without stress. Everyone should learn how to take it and live with it. If this seems impossible, you are in the wrong place or working at the wrong job. Drugs cannot remedy stress and strain. Coffee and tea should be taken sparingly, drugs and tranquilizers only in emergencies, and cigarettes not at all. These so-called "aids" can become trouble-makers, forming unhealthly habits subject to disagreeable side effects. Coffee and alcohol are digestive destroyers. Coffee drinking can also bring on heart failure, tension, and impaired memory.

The health troubles of today are multiplied by articles of convenience. Elevators do away with stairs walking. Automobiles deprive the average person of using his or her own legs for moving about. The use of a second telephone in the home prevents the housewife from getting the exercise her body needs.

Most mature men have trouble with their arteries. If the average businessman today were to race a hundred yards, he might drop dead before reaching his goal. That is the state of what might be called "business health" today. Dr. White frowned upon the idea of human heart transplants. He dislikes any temporary expedience. Although many intricate mechanical devices have been brought into existence to replace certain organs in the body, real lasting success has not been achieved, though they have extended the lives of some people temporarily.

COLON TROUBLES —

My work in aiding ailing folks through the years has convinced me positively that all bodily disease generates in the colon. The reason for this is that the colon is the collective dumping ground for the waste material from the digestive organs. Much of the modern food that is eaten is not properly digested because of the lack of enzymes in the food which have been killed by heat, etc. Should this debris not be eliminated from the body within a limited time, it rots, gases form, and it becomes a breeding ground for harmful bacteria. These germs set up housekeeping in the weakest spots of the body and in these spots disease starts to flourish under various names. The toxins and poison formed in the colon gradually work their way into the bloodstream and cause pollution of this precious life line. This contamination many times overtaxes the liver and weakens the kidneys. Most persons with cancer, as a result suffer liver weaknesses.

Fortunes have been spent on cancer research with very little attention paid to investigation of the fertile field where cancer has its start—*the colon*. The reason that the colon is the seat of cancer is because the cooked food has had its valuable enzymes destroyed by heat. Also, many mixtures of food combinations prevents the proper digestive activities from operating in a normal way. Eating too often interferes seriously with digestive processes. When a person puts more food in the stomach before the material eaten previously has been adequately taken care of complications result. Overeating also puts too much additional strain upon the digestive system, thus causing constipation. Tension also can prevent the proper digestion of food. Of course, deficiencies in the food eaten may cause mental disorders. Mother Nature needs materials to repair nerves, etc. Experience has demonstrated that victims of illnesses are usually constipated and have serious colon congestions. This condition should receive careful attention.

Unfortunately, few folks realize the very important function underlying good digestion. These underlying functions are easy to understand. Normal digestion depends primarily upon food that has been thoroughly chewed and mixed with saliva before swallowing. The start of the digestive processes originates in the mouth. Thus, when the food reaches the stomach, it is easily acted upon by the hydrochloric acid and the juices from the pancreas. The bile from the liver aids further. Food improperly chewed, ferments in the colon and gases form. Especially this is true of all starches and fats. This emphasizes the need of having all factors of the digestive system working normally. This is true especially when the liver is not working as it should and is unable to separate out the impurities. Disfunction of the liver enables toxins to enter the bloodstream bringing on old age and sickness.

The colon is the depository of waste material, after the essentials from the food have been extracted and have entered the bloodstream where they feed the cells which help to maintain health and keep the body active and young. The waste from the colon should be eliminated as often as food is taken into the body. If this is not done, the decaying food rots and breeds parasites. Therefore, the clogged colon is the body's disease breeding place. All ailments and disease start in the colon and it is the colon which should demand our first attention in every health emergency.

There are many causes for cancer but the main trouble is some deficiency in the diet. Also, the body may be unable to remove the waste from the bloodstream due to weaknesses in the digestive organs. Generally in such instances the kidneys and liver are overlooked. This is the reason they were unable to do their alloted tasks properly. Most important of all is the condition of the colon. It is the breeding ground for cancer when constipation takes over.

The debris in the colon forms gases and these gases are distributed through the lymphatic system throughout the body. Of course, as every human body has some weakness somewhere, these gases find a suitable starting point. There is a definite solution and it is a simple solution that is most effective and economical to handle the cancer problem. Cleanse the bloodstream and give the blood that opportunity to rebuild the cells properly. As I said before, chlorophyll is the only way to solve the colon problem.

MENTAL ILLNESS —

Malnutrition is at last being recognized as a major cause of mental illness. A chemical imbalance in the brain caused by malnutrition has been described by Dr. Linus Pauling in his article on Orthomolecular Psychiatry. Despite these documented facts, Dr. Pauling was severely criticized for having no evidence to substantiate his views. Dr. Pauling answered, "My associate and I have carried on research on the molecular basis of mental diseases for twelve years. For ten of those years, I have been aware of the opposition of many psychiatrists to the idea that patients might benefit by having a supply of vitamins and nutrients different from that recommended for the average patient."

The mentally ill patient has a more acute need for proper nutrition than the average patient. Much mental illness could be prevented and some could be cured by proper nutrition. So long as patients are fed white bread, white sugar, hydrogenated fats, refined salt and overprocessed cereals, our mental hospitals will remain filled. While drug treatment of mental illness may suppress the symptons, the prevention and cure depend upon proper nutrition. Since no psychiatrist would suggest that proper nutrition might harm a mentally ill person, it is at least worth a try. As Dr. Pauling has said, ". . . a psychiatrist who refuses to try the methods of orthomolecular psychiatry (understood as proper nutrition) in addition to the usual therapy in treatment of his patients is failing in his duty as a physician."

FEAR —

During my years of experience in helping the very sick, I have learned that every serious affliction is aggravated by fear. Fear prevents healing. Worry is a great obstacle to health, and even in these times when there seems to be so much to worry about, a natural program of living helps alleviate worries of all kinds. Our newspapers tell us that hospital costs will soon rise to $300 per day and that doctors will be highly paid "specialists". We must acquire a completely new outlook, physically, mentally and spiritually. When the body improves physically, fear vanishes and the mentality is guided to a clear understanding of the laws of God. A spark of God is in all human beings, animals and plants. This spark should be given every chance to mature naturally.

TIREDNESS —

Stimulants are used almost universally to keep the body moving. Many business executives are now using drugs during office hours to find the energies their positions require. Doctors Lanley and Margison have made extensive studies in this field and have found that dope is common on Wall Street. We find that when we deal with employees of large organizations, we are frequently met with listlessness, indifference, and lack of understanding. Amphetamines are used extensively by workers who lack the natural engeries to keep up with the work required of them. Many of these employees are in fact sick and this sickness often stems from lack of proper nourishment.

Unaccountable bone deep weariness is a definite signal that all is not well with the delicate internal machinery of the body. German investigator Dr. Otto Warburg demonstrated that poisons in the system interfere with the enzyme system which carries oxygen to the cells and enables our cells to utilize the nutrients in the food we eat. *TODAY'S HEALTH* informs its readers that without enzymes man cannot digest his food, breathe, move muscles, reproduce, or perform any of his body's functions normally. Cells may be irreparably damaged to such an extent that the body is reduced to as little as one-seventh of its normal efficiency. The essential first step is to change our eating habits. Uncooked foods, containing the little "spark plugs" of enzymes, should be eaten to awaken the tiring cells to new life. Living food is the substance which gives us vitality and keeps us healthy and youthful.

People have arrived at the Hippocrates Health Institute from the four corners of the earth, bringing with them all types of common miseries: diabetes, asthma, allergies, headaches, constipation, psoriasis, emphysema, high and low blood pressure, arthritis, bursitis, ulcers, gall stones and kidney stones, leukemia, eye problems, catarrh, rheumatism, overweight, colitis, emotional upsets, digestive disturbances, polio, cancer and a host of other afflictions.

God has created in every body a wondrous, self-sustaining, self-regulating, self-healing mechanism. Twenty-five hundred years ago, Hippocrates said, "Let food be thy medicine." Hippocrates theorized that it was necessary to first remove the cause of bodily upset and then to provide Nature with the proper tools to repair the damage. These tools included a semi-fast to cleanse the bloodstream, food to bring live nourishment to the cells, moist heat and massage to relax the muscles, clean air to bring oxygen to the lungs, exercise to stimulate the circulation, fresh water to lubricate the body tissues, and the dismissal of all fear to permit real relaxation.

Through the years, extensive experiments have been performed, feeding living, uncooked, organically grown food to both human beings and animals, many miracles of health improvement have come to light. These accomplishments prove the absolute truth of Hippocrates saying that "food should be the medicine of all human beings and animals."

At the Hippocrates Health Institute, we teach the laws of Mother Nature. We are showing how one can help a degenerated body regain health and youth. When folks understand Mother Nature's methods and follow her fundamental laws, the wonderful inner glow of good health results. Such healthy folks are generally eager to lead others to health by their example. We learn that through helping others, we help ourselves. We add treasures to our own happiness and are energized by the feeling of accomplishment.

DOCTORS
MEDICAL and NATURAL

Perfect health is the birthright of all living things. Wild animals in their natural environment are never sick. According to the Hebrew scribes, the average life span of human beings should be one thousand years, as it was in ancient times when humans were guided by instinct to select proper nourishment. It is about time we made some open-minded investigations of the present conditions in the civilized world regarding health. Nothing just happens. There is a definite reason for all bodily upsets.

Since Hippocrates' era, the medical profession has flourished. It has perfected miraculous methods to alleviate pain. Yet many so-called short cuts, though they may offer immediate relief, actually foster serious and lasting side effects and may promote chronic ill health far worse than the original upset. Many dedicated physicians fully realize the shortcomings of strong drugs and are seriously concerned about their side effects. Dr. Herbert Ratner, Director of Public Health and Professor of Medicine at Loyola University Medical School, calls America "the most over-medicated, most over-inoculated country in the world." We have earned the disgraceful reputation of the "sickest nation on earth."

Doctors know that drug therapy is secondary to proper nourishment, exercise, rest and relaxation. Medical doctors hold the public confidence and are in the strongest position to advocate living, uncooked food. However, the simplicity of natural healing mitigates against its wide acceptance. Although physicians realize that the underlying cause of illness must be eliminated before normal health can resume, those who have spent arduous years perfecting their professional abilities do not appreciate quick and easy methods.

It is most unfortunate that folks everywhere are seeking "cures" without any effort to remove the cause of their condition. When the human body sickens from the chemicalized nutrition it receives today, more poison is added to the body in the form of drugs and injections in an effort to regain normal health. These so-called "medicines" create side effects and raise additional health problems. Many persons fear the pathogenic bacteria that may invade the body and seek to kill the invaders with antibiotic drugs, believing such acts will prevent disaster. These frightened people do not realize that to destroy the harmful germs, one must also exterminate the beneficial ones, the little workers who toil tirelessly, repairing, reconditioning, healing and defending our health. The sober truth is that there is no cure for anything besides the body's inherent ability to heal itself. However, it must receive our cooperation to achieve success.

The human bloodstream is the sacred vehicle of life and must be kept well-nourished and clean. When your body is healthy, it is not prone to disease. Weak points, where germs set up housekeeping, are eliminated. Invading germs seek some type of rubbish heap, toxin-laden cells where the environment is satisfactory for their growth. Digestive tracts clogged with a myriad of prescriptions, cathartics, aspirin and other pain killers and drugs, provide that environment. A wise doctor once said, "The only sickness which exists in the body is toxicity. Healthy cells, nourished properly with organic living food, are immune from such attacks."

The "outside" painkiller is against all the laws of Nature. A painkiller, even under the best circumstances, gives the body a shock that effects every organ and tissue. The entire delicate mechanism is thrown off balance and the effects of that disturbance may make themselves known physically and mentally actually months later.

It was the researcher Dr. G. H. Earp-Thomas whose delicate experiments with many types of animals made him certain that even a mild painkiller leaves its effects on the internal mechanism. As he once remarked to me, "A single aspirin, which the average doctor hands out to sufferers with no more thought than if they were sugar pills, often causes brain damage that the body might be unable to rectify during its lifetime." I am in close agreement with his conclusion because of the damaged mentalities I have had to encounter during the past several years. Most of the mental problems I have faced have had their foundations in the utilization of aspirin as a starter. When these so-called mild drugs seem to fail in their purpose after fairly long periods of use, they prove to be a mere stepping stone to some harsher type of dope which eventually turns the user into a helpless addict, unable to break the chains of habit.

Under the powerful microscope of Dr. Earp-Thomas, I saw ordinary helpful bacteria, which moved about in the drop of liquid, begin to slow down and actually become stationary when a little piece of aspirin pill, reduced to powder form, was added to the liquid. Under the same microscope some six hours later, that single drop was stagnant and dead. What happened to that liquid is happening to many of the tissues supplied by the lymphatic system of the body when almost any type of the so-called "harmless" painkillers is introduced into the body.

Most medical doctors do not look upon such disturbances with alarm. They seem to believe that the positive electricity of the body can right matters in due time and no permanent scars will be left. They follow the theory of the physician who vaccinates the human being and calmly informs the victim that he is "probably immune for the next ten years", without disclosing the fact that the poisonous substance he introduced into the patient's bloodstream would float around in the body and the blood for that length of time before it would be thrown out of the body.

The October, 1971, issue of the *The New News,* reports that the State of France was required to pay indemnity to a young girl who was a victim of a smallpox vaccination and damages to her parents. The Court also ruled against the Inspector of the Academy of Vanes who refused entrance in the school to children not vaccinated, even though they had certificates of contre-indication. Dr. J. Spencer, the Chief of the Control of Contagious Diseases, applauded the decision of the Minister of Health to stop smallpox vaccinations of the masses, believing that the reactions to the vaccination are more often dangerous than the illness. For twenty years, he explained, no person at E.U.A. has contracted this illness, but numerous accidents, with six deaths, from the vaccination is registered. Since 1970, this certificate is no longer required from persons entering E.U.A. except travellers from Pakistan, India, Afghanistan, Ethiopia, and Sudan, where smallpox still exists.

The human bloodstream is a closed circuit. The Almighty made it so. Everything that goes into the blood in a natural way must pass through the intricate natural filters which keep out dangerous substances. The medical man, with his hypodermic needle, bypasses these protective filters and the bloodstreams are polluted by thousands, setting up countless weak spots for ill health to start. Painkillers are extremely dangerous. They have no rightful place in our Holy Temples.

Although millions of dollars are spent each year on the study of eliminating disease, practically nothing has been done until recently to teach the average person the way of maintaining good health and to eliminate disease through the use of living, uncooked food. We are now approaching a breakthrough in this work which will benefit laymen and doctors alike. Many orthodox physicians, chiropractors, osteopaths, physical therapists, ministers and social workers have adopted our live foods program. They have experienced it to be effective treatment for ill health, inexpensive and universally available. This development will not only make living more enjoyable for the average person, but will also lengthen the lives of the doctors themselves.

More and more doctors are turning their attention to diet and are appreciating the virtues of living food and the effect it has upon the health of the body. They are handing out diets instead of drug store prescriptions. And they are beginning to understand that prescriptions, while aimed at one particular spot in the body, have many side effects that drag down, rather than improve, bodily health.

No one healing method is self-sufficient. A chiropractor can realign a displaced spine; an osteopath can uncongest stiff ligaments; a physical therapist can relax bodily tension. And a spiritual healer can purify our mentality, uplift our spirit. Yoga keeps us young and flexible. Astrology helps us better understand ourselves. We develop health through all of Nature's avenues.

Health begins with faith. Faith in God, without Whom we can achieve nothing. Faith in His system; faith in our bodies. Jesus said, "If you can but understand as I understand, you can heal yourself." That means that if you have faith, your spirit, which is never ill, can so direct your body that it will become perfect as the Almighty intended it to be. If ailments plague and trouble a person, it is because the house of that spirit, the human body, merely is being used in the wrong way. Sickness is caused by neglect, ignorance and the direct abuse of the body through harmful habits and deficient foods. Wild animals, ruled by instinct, have no harmful habits and are never ill. If human beings were guided today entirely by instinct alone, there would be no sickness among us. Spiritual healing brings the body back under the fixed laws of God.

My experience in working with ailing human beings has shown me that faith healing is very essential in these trying times. The person who lives more on the physical plane has a much harder time. Such a person lacks the mental belief that help is coming, which is so essential to recovery. We should have the feeling that nothing is impossible. Every idea which seems right should be coupled with the thought that nothing can prevent its being carried through if we seek God's help.

No thought works out by itself. Physical effort is necessary in order to put ideas into practice. With utmost patience and unalterable faith, one must await and accept guidance from within. When we meditate for a solution to our problem, we are informing God of our needs. If the answers are not forthcoming, the fault lies with us alone. If our mind is clear and our plan true, there is no need for concern. When we seek God's aid, we need patience, understanding, wisdom and freedom from prejudice. Our faith can equip us to meet any challenge and guide us to a satisfying answer.

Circumstances have shown me that God placed each one of us here on earth for a definite purpose. We may be guided by an intuitive urge to do whatever is essential to fulfill this purpose. There now exists a God-given opportunity to bring to suffering humanity the outstanding healthful advantages of living food. To become a Healing Scientist, the most important thing is to become a worthy example to others, to live the Gospel. In order to do this, we have to give up many old ideas and habits. If we ask God's help, He will give us the strength and will power. We must always remember that we are co-workers with God, that thoughts are things and will manifest eventually whatever we have put forth, either good or bad. The Healing Scientist should always look upon everything that happens with a loving and understanding attitude. Such a viewpoint will always lead to victory.

There is a place for both the orthodox medical man and the natural physican. The skills of both augment the abilities of each and make their work with suffering humanity progressively better. The orthodox doctors and the natural healing practitioners should study each other's methods. A minister of the Gospel should also be a physician. Likewise, an orthodox physician should be familiar with spiritual healing. Treating the body and the soul at the same time is essential for the regaining of lost health. A discouraged soul drags the body down, while an alert mentality speeds recovery. Proper nourishment is the "open sesame", the only way to health.

Part II

Wheatgrass— God's Manna

THE DISCOVERY

Our simple remedy for helping people is the God-given chlorophyll of the wheatgrass. Nature uses it as a body cleanser, rebuilder and neutralizer of toxin. The effectiveness of chlorophyll, derived from fresh wheatgrass juice and sprouts of various grains and seeds, is under study at many important research institutions. Dr. G. H. Earp-Thomas, scientist and soil expert, isolated over one hundred elements from fresh wheatgrass and concluded that it is a complete food. Fifteen pounds of fresh wheatgrass is equivalent in nutritional value to 350 pounds of the choicest vegetables.

Charles Kettering of General Motors has been donating $30,000 each year to Antioch College for the study of chlorophyll as a healing agent. Dr. Fisher, a Nobel Prize winner, used chlorophyll to treat anemia. The American Journal of Surgery, July, 1940, reported twelve hundred cases of peritonitis, brain ulcer, pyorrhea and skin disorders cured by chlorophyll.

Dr. Richard Willstater observed that the chlorophyll molecule bears close resemblance to hemoglobin, the red pigment in human blood, and differs only in the central element which in blood is iron and in chlorophyll magnesium. Owing to their close molecular resemblance, it was believed by Frans Miller, another scientist, that chlorophyll is the natural blood building element for all plant eaters and humans. He writes, "Chlorophyll has the same fast blood building effects as iron in animals made experimentally anemic."

Dr. Birscher, a research scientist, called chlorophyll "concentrated sun power." He said, "Chlorophyll increases the function of the heart, effects the vascular system, the intestines, the uterus, and the lungs. It raises the basic nitrogen exchange and is therefore a tonic which, considering its stimulating properties, cannot be compared with any other."

At Temple University, Doctors Gurskin, Redpath and Davis used chlorophyll to successfully treat over one thousand patients for all forms of ear, nose and throat problems. Dr. Carroll Wright found chlorophyll effective on chronic ulcers.

Some 120 centuries ago, on the continent of Atlantis, it was predicted that the real health-giving properties of wheatgrass would be learned by some far distant generation, when men would be given the key to save a tottering civilization from extinction. We believe that we have found this key.

The Discovery—

In a remote section of war-torn Europe where bloody hand-to-hand encounters between Russians and Germans occupied two solid nightmarish years, I came to know the most wonderful physician in the world—my grandmother. Only God could have given her the knowledge she bestowed everywhere. Resourceful, kind and compassionate she was the unnamed leader of the few remaining villagers who huddled waistdeep in the water in the root cellar of our shell-blasted orchard. Our provisions gone, we gnawed bark from the tree roots which had pushed through the walls and chewed grass my grandmother brought back from her ghost-like forays into the hellish nights. But rising water soon made our shelter a graveyard. So grandmother led the flight for life across the open field as bullets zipped past our ears. Some fell, and we dodged the prostrate forms like frightened children. Of that terrible drawnout ordeal, I most vividly recall the grass which brought me, a frail sickly child, through alive.

When I arrived in the United States, I was in my teens. I had lived under rather hazardous conditions for a decade and, like those around me, had suffered from insufficient food. I had dined more or less regularly on roots, grass and rough bread composed of rye meal and straw, with the emphasis on the straw. When I arrived in Middleboro, Massachusetts, I had perfect, strong teeth, but within twelve months of consuming coca-cola, doughnuts and other refined foods, I was forced to have four of my back teeth extracted. The dentist admitted that the wonderful American foods lacked the necessary nutritional elements of the rough diet of Europe.

My health, which had been poor since birth, was failing in the New World. Because the physicians and drugstores seemed powerless to help me, I instinctively turned to God for guidance. I began to study my Bible and I recall, as though it were only yesterday, that afternoon in my room with the warm sunshine streaming past the edges of the drawn curtain, when these simple words came to me: "Become a minister and build my temples." That moment brought me, a much puzzled girl, to the wondrous path I have followed ever since. Preparing myself for the ministry was not easy. My meager education consisted of knowledge I had acquired from nature as a sheepherder and assistant to my grandmother in her care of the suffering and dying during those dreadful war days of the First World War. When the goal of my ministry was finally in sight, the realization of what God had meant by "build my temples" came to me one winter's morning. I saw clearly that the temples I was commissioned to build were God's most precious creations, human bodies - "The Temples of the Soul."

Not until I became a resident of Boston, living across the street from the Christian Science Cathedral, was the "how" of building or rebuilding these temples shown to me. In the Book of Daniel, Fourth Chapter, in the Old Testament, I read of the sick king who, heeding the voice from heaven, went into the field and "eating grass as did the oxen", regained his physical and mental health. If grass could completely rebuild the decrepit body of King Nebuchadnezzar, I reasoned, it could today rebuild the tottering bodies I saw all around me.

I quickly discovered, however, that grasses differ both in structure and value and are comprised of more than 350 divisions, divided into 4700 species, from the one-hundred-foot towering bamboo of the tropics to the inch high, threadlike grass of the artic tundra. Ordinary grass, I learned, afforded a six hundred pound steer sufficient carotene and Vitamin A for all nutritious purposes with an abundance of riboflavin, nicotinic and panthothenic acids. But I had to have the best and most nutritious grass available.

Despite the pessimistic predictions of friends, I wrote letters to hundreds of health students around the world, begging them to send me samples of their native grasses. Within a matter of weeks, I received seeds from the four corners of the earth: bluegrass from Kentucky, pampas grass from the Argentine, tree grass from Australia, etc. All these I planted separately and watched for the signs soil experts had recommended: rapid growth, widespread roots, sturdy stalks, and quick evidence of chlorophyll, the grass juice. At the end of my watch, seven grasses qualified: Rye, Timothy, Broome, Wheat, Canary, Alfalfa and Buckwheat. The question arose in my mind: Should I mix the seeds of the seven grasses and use the miscellaneous blades together, or should I select one grass at random? I would let God guided creatures decide.

Next morning, refreshed from a good night's sleep, I had my answer. In a room where I could follow the proceedings unobserved, I arranged my seven small pots of grass. Into this room I placed a small kitten. I watched as the kitten went and sniffed each a wisp of grass before finally choosing the wheatgrass to chew. But I wanted more proof. From a friend I borrowed a little cocker spaniel. Like the kitten, it too chose the wheatgrass. There could be no doubt. Wheatgrass was the grass I sought.

The next step was to try the wheatgrass juice on my own body. Months of patient testing followed. My shattered health experienced miraculous recovery. Where before I was unable to work for but a few hours a day because of exhaustion and nervousness, the wheatgrass seemed to bring new alertness and energy into my body. No task seemed to be too difficult to accomplish and work became a pleasure instead of a chore. I even began to feel younger, and I realized, probably for the first time, that wheatgrass is a God-send and had arrived at the right time to change the chemistry of my blood, enabling me to survive those difficult times.

Friends who had confidence in me agreed to try it. Without exception all told of more alertness, freedom from pain, peaceful sleep, and longer working hours spent undisturbed by tired muscles or drowsiness. Still I was not satisfied. I wanted scientific assay of the worth of wheatgrass chlorophyll by a distinguished and highly experienced agriculturist. Probably the foremost soil expert in the world at that time was Dr. G. H. Earp-Thomas of New Jersey. For more than half a century, his investigations had been helping agriculturists all over the world contribute to satisfying the food needs of the earth's expanding population. I had known him slightly for a time and when I appeared in his laboratory and told him my story, I found him most sympathetic. It was the first of my many visits to his office and the beginning of an exciting adventure into unforeseen realms.

Through a microscope I learned about the world of tiny organisms that lived unnoticed in all good soil. I learned that certain bacteria must be present in fertile soil to destroy alien forms of life. I learned that nature only cherishes healthy vegetation and ruthlessly destroys every vestige of growth that does not meet her standards of excellence. I learned that chemical fertilizers denature natural growth. While chemicals temporarily bring forth oversized vegetation, they ultimately wipe out all evidence of life and create a desert unsuitable for living organisms.

Next came more experiments. I separated six-day old chicks into two groups of three chicks each. Each group was fed the best acceptable type of chick feed. But in one cage I mixed chopped up, freshly gathered wheatgrass with the food and placed a sprig of wheatgrass in the drinking water. At the end of a few weeks, all the chicks were healthy, but those receiving the wheatgrass had grown twice as large as the others. They were more alert and had feathered out better. Groups of rabbits and kittens, fed in similar fashion, showed the same results in size, weight and mentality.

I knew then that I had been entrusted with a precious secret to help people. Over the years, I have worked fervently to make this secret known. Now others are experimenting and discovering the wondrous benefits of wheatgrass. Years of experience have proven conclusively that wheatgrass therapy is fundamentally sound. We need only to look to the fields and forests to learn from the wild animals. They have no hospitals, no doctors, no medicine, yet they are ruled by the same laws of creation that govern humans. If a wild animal feels sick, it will instinctively fast or nibble grass.

The Bible says that each one of us is made of the "dust" of the Earth; and as 103 known elements make up this world, somewhere in every well human body is every one of these 103 elements, some doubtlessly utilized only in the amount of a single grain. Yet if that is missing, sickness results. Hippocrates said, "Into man there enters a breath, having a blend of fire (sunlight) and water, a portion of man's body. These are nourished and increased by human diet. Now the things that enter must contain all the parts." The only food which seems to contain all 103 nutriments is grass, which is the only food which will healthfully support an animal from birth to prime old age. And human beings, in the final analysis, are the highest form of animals.

Over twenty-four hundred years ago, Hippocrates wisely said, "Let food be thy medicine." In this simple declaration is summed up the experience of not only Hippocrates but many researchers of his time who were seeking fundamental tenets of human existence. His food-therapy principle is incorporated completely in the wheatgrass therapy. Through the modern conception and use of this ancient idea, bodily upsets, acute and chronic, have been miraculously corrected. Thousands of our students, in their homes, without expert supervision, have proven conclusively that proper nutrition is more than a match for ill health. When such a disorder becomes manifest, it indicates ignorance or carelessness on the part of the victim. Wild animals, in their native environment are rarely sick, yet domesticated animals, cared for and fed by man, are seldom well. Wild animals select their food through instinct alone and make few mistakes. Domesticated animals must eat what humans feed them and consequently they suffer from a multitude of disorders.

Wheatgrass is not a "cure". However, through scientific investigation and experimentation, we have discovered that it furnishes the body with vital nourishment, which, when missing, yields sickness and disease. Since scores of physicians are certain that ingesting reasonable amounts of wheatgrass juice will not complicate any existing ailments, common sense indicates that we test its miraculous possibilities on your own bodies. Many physicians here in Boston have tested the miraculous effectiveness of the wheatgrass therapy. They have proven to their own satisfaction that wheatgrass chlorophyll is a New Age food—medicine capable of alleviating the problems of sick humanity. Come to the Hippocrates Health Institute to learn how we can become our own doctors. Let's cut our medical bills and banish our worries about ill health. Start a new life by claiming our birthright—good health.

THE
ROAD TO HEALTH
THE
WHEATGRASS FAST

You have prayed for guidance and now you are ready to put that guidance into action. Anyone who comes to the Mansion for help should be determined to undertake the wheatgrass fast for seven days. Total fasting is not recommended. While it is true that total fasting allows the body to cleanse itself of accumulated poisons, the further elimination of food from the already undernourished victim may severely complicate his health problems. We have found the ideal solution in the wheatgrass fast which countless individuals have undertaken without harm. This fast provides the body with all the nutrients of the richest living food in a form so concentrated and easy to digest that it provides virtually all the benefits of a complete fast with none of the dangers of total abstinence. Such a fast can pleasantly cleanse and nourish at the same time. One can be confident of complete safety and real health building results.

In preparation for the fast, it is sound practice to undergo a colonic irrigation to clean out the body. Food which accumulates in the walls of the intestines over the years decomposes, creating impurities, poisons, and toxins. It is necessary to eliminate this putrefection. Check your yellow pages to find the nearest establishment where this treatment is given.

Because every human being differs in body and thought, fasting cannot be undertaken successfully on an assembly line basis. Similarly, the duration of the fast should be expertly determined on the basis of the individual's actual needs. The wheatgrass fast consists of three or four wheatgrass juice drinks each day plus two chlorophyll implants. If your body rebels against the taste or odor of the juice, the same results may be obtained by taking four implants instead of two.

Upon awakening, drink two glasses of warm water with the juice of one lemon added. This drink may be sweetened with molasses or honey. Then the colon should be throughly evacuated with an enema to eliminate any debris clinging to the inner walls of the colon. Four ounces of the pure wheatgrass chlorophyll should be sipped three times a day at well spaced intervals. Each drink may be diluted with as much water as is desired. The faster should drink at least one quart of not-too-cold water each day, placing a wisp of wheatgrass in each drink to purify it. Cold water may delay the digestive action of the stomach and intestines for several hours.

I have found one may experience weakness during the wheatgrass fast on one day or more. The quickest and most effective way to meet this crisis is to drink sesame milk. This drink is high in protein and calcium and should alleviate the sense of weakness. If you feel that you must eat, use grapes or watermelon in season. If for any reason you must interrupt your fast, set aside an evening for a small meal of mung, alfalfa, or lentil sprouts, or a salad of green, leafy vegetables, and then return to the fast.

As you begin to tread this natural path, do not be surprised when your body begins to awaken to the changes. Those who lose weight only with difficulty will find that the wheatgrass fast, if followed faithfully, will eliminate at least one-half pound every twenty-four hours. To those overweight individuals who frequently experience digestive disorders, the wheatgrass fast permits their digestive systems a much needed rest. Once you have started your wheatgrass fast, the chlorophyll will bring toxins stored away in cells or in fatty tissue into the bloodstream. This cleansing action may be accompanied by nausea, headaches, fever and cramps. Do not be alarmed. Simply lie down and rest until you feel better. Some people find relief by chewing a little celery. Plenty of rest is vital during this cleansing period to enable your body to divest itself of the toxic accumulations of a lifetime of wrong eating, medications and other abuses.

WHEATGRASS IMPLANTS —

The implants of wheatgrass chlorophyll constitute the greatest blood cleanser and builder known. The wheatgrass chlorophyll is very rapidly assimilated by the body because its composition is similar to the hemoglobin molecule in the blood. It can actually save human life when oral feeding is impossible. The colon is cleansed simultaneously. I am certain that most health problems begin in the colon. Generally, meat eaters develop worms, and these blood destroyers reside in the colon during the entire life of the victim. They sap energy and cause fever, constipation, and a host of other problems.

For your wheatgrass implants, you need a regular enema bag, not the combination kind. You also need an eighteen inch catheter to replace the usual rectal tube. The glass connecting unit comes with the catheter.

When you take your enema with warm water, be sure to treat the water with wheatgrass to counteract possible chemicals. You may insert the catheter completely into your rectum. The best position for an enema is to lie flat on the floor on your left side. If you have any difficulty retaining all the water, breathe deeply through your mouth. To massage the abdomen while the water is implanted, which is also beneficial, move your hand in a clockwise, circular motion. The ascending colon is on the right, so this spot should be massaged upward in your motion.

Another method to remove the debris from the colon is to lie flat on your back, put your legs in the air and ride an imaginary bicycle. Some people prefer to take enemas on the floor resting on their knees and chest. Others will want to use the usual slant board. Each person must learn his own best method for taking enemas. We are all individual and no set method is applicable to all for best results. Colonics are also suitable if the person prefers them.

It is best to wait about one-half hour after an enema before implanting the chlorophyll. The chlorophyll is implanted like an ordinary water enema and must be retained in the body for twenty to thirty minutes to gain the maximum benefit.

However, do not hold either enema or implant for longer than thirty minutes or dissolved waste materials will be reabsorbed into the bloodstream. It is best to begin with half a cup and increase to a cup by easy stages. I find it helpful for difficulty in retaining the chlorophyll to lie on my back and brace my feet against the wall or some object such as a bed, wash bowl, etc. Be sure to press the anus with tissue paper and if we feel any gas, allow it to escape. Above all, we must never dread this important health function. Such fear tenses us and interferes with the whole process. Breathe deeply through the mouth to relax. While we are holding our implant, we can practice spot therapy on our feet to loosen up toxic spots; also massage our face and scalp.

For active persons, it is easiest to take the implant in the evening. Should we decide to have two implants a day, we must be sure to take them about two hours apart while the colon is still clean. These steps will not only help us feel and look younger, but will also prevent sickness. Above all, never give up. Keep trying; practice makes prefect.

A Word For Bedridden "Incurables" —

I receive many letters and long distance telephone calls pleading for help when some loved one has been cast out of the hospital as hopeless and has been sent home to die. Most of these people are helplessly bedridden, unable to aid themselves. It is heartbreaking when I am forced to tell the anxious family or relatives that I cannot accept them to the Mansion since we have no nurses or attendants. In order to help those who seek aid in such circumstances, the following suggestions should prove helpful.

Watch The Elimination —

This is very important. Relieve constipation with enemas, colonics or massage. Daily sponge baths of warm water are essential. These should be followed by a body rub with a rough cloth to help circulation.

Soaking the feet in warm water for fifteen or twenty minutes each day helps to eliminate the poisons from the system that gravity has pulled down to the feet and ankles. It also aids in relaxation. Massage is also helpful, though the person giving the massage should be in good physical condition as the health vibrations pass from the masseur's body adding strength and vitality to the weaker one. Massaging the cords in the back and sides of the neck strengthens the mentality of the ailing person. Wriggling the toes for several minutes, morning and night, is also helpful.

When a person is bedridden, *liquid food* is the best type of nourishment. No matter how good the food is, if it cannot be properly digested, it will turn into poisons causing gas and other discomforts. Live nourishment, uncooked, starves the diseased organisms and strengthens the health bacteria. No acid fruits should be taken as the body is already too acidy. Baked food and bread should be avoided. Wheatgrass juice should be taken or implanted in the colon. Crushed and strained watermelon juice is alkaline and easily digestible. Fresh coconut milk is acceptable and when small bits of fresh coconut are blended with an equal amount of water, strained and flavored with a little maple syrup, it has in many instances proven to be a successful addition to the diet and a delicious drink. A sesame seed drink, blended and strained, is a good source of protein, if it can be tolerated. Wheat milk is also beneficial as is the live juice from raw vegetables and mild fruit. A book on live juices may be purchased at your local health store.

Rejuvalac is a new form of acidophilus made from soaking one cup of wheat in two cups of water for twenty-four hours. This is a superior form of digestive culture which aids the very ill. Two or three glasses of rejuvalac can be taken each day. Because this drink improves digestion, persons who were underweight have been able to gain extra pounds.

Remember, each person is different. What is agreeable to one may not be to another. Give to the sick what they respond to best. Realize wholeheartedly that with God nothing is impossible. He often performs miracles for bettered health despite the pessimistic prediction of the experts. Mother Nature is more than willing to help if she is provided with the proper tools. Keep up your faith and your efforts. Always be cheerful and relaxed when working with your loved one. Think positively. Because the sufferer must depend on you for all his needs, he becomes very sensitive to your moods.

TESTIMONIALS

"My Dear Dr. Wigmore,

I would be remiss if I didn't let you and the whole world know how much I learned and benefited from your lessons and guidance in the field of nutrition and its relation to Live Foods. I had the extreme pleasure of hearing you lecture at the National Health Federation Convention at the Hotel New Yorker a few years ago, and it was the turning point in my life. The reasons which I will explain in the latter part of my letter.

I am a graduate of a college and a university namely New York University. At both schools, I specialized in Health Education, which included a number of courses of Hygiene, the study of the care of the body. I have been a teacher of Health Education in the New York City high schools since 1934. That which I learned in college was purely academic, that is, anatomy and physiology. In the area of meaningful and informative nutrition, very little was taught.

To get back to the first paragraph. You have taught me practical hygiene. You have taught me how I could supply the body's nutritional needs for pennies a day. You have taught me how to raise my food in my own kitchen by sprouting. How I can live on organically fertilized food free from sprays. You have taught me how to make wheat "milk" which is superior to cow's milk. You have taught me how important uncooked food is and under your patient guidance I dismissed all fears and doubts. I replace them with faith and confidence, working with Mother Nature.

I am sixty-six years of age and am still very active in school gymnasium work. I demonstrate daily on the parallel bars, horse, high bar, ropes and weights. I am also engaged in a daily exercise and sports program as is required in my work.

As I told you frankly, I gained more practical health knowledge at the Mansion than I did at the two colleges from which I was graduated. This should be the age of prevention rather than the treatment of ills. You certainly are a beacon of hope in a land of ignorance and miseducation in the area of health.

I cannot repay you ever for what you have done for me and my family. Bless you."   M. H.   Brooklyn, N.Y.

ARTHRITIS —

"An attorney, knowing my husband was troubled pain-fully with arthritis, gave him a copy of *Why Suffer?* We both read the book and were so impressed that we had an indoor garden of wheatgrass growing within two days. My husband began taking it as soon as it was five inches tall. We cut down on our eating—trying to follow your simple diet. The results were miraculous. Getting up in the morning no longer meant massage and groans. After just seven days on your therapy, he was able to tie his own shoes without help. Within two weeks, on two drinks a day, morning and evening, his pains and the swollen redness about the knees disappeared."

R. M.   Michigan

ASTHMA —

"For many, many years I was a sufferer with asthma. And every so often my husband would have to rush me to the hospital in an ambulance where I would stay in the oxygen tank. I seemed to be allergic to everything. Especially in the Spring, I would have the hardest kind of time to live.

A friend gave me your literature and I did not waste time to make the trip to the Mansion. I stayed on there three weeks. But in that time, my asthma completely disappeared. At that time you were doing some experiments with little chicks. They did not bother me one bit, though on former occasions they made me breathless. My friends tell me I look twenty years younger and now I am back to work once more, which I was forced to give up because of my health.

"When I visited my doctor, he warned me that I would have the asthma again. That was three years ago, and since that trouble did not arrive, he certainly cannot understand why I am very, very grateful to you for giving me new life."

G. A.   Massachusetts

BE YOUR OWN DOCTOR —

"I cannot begin to tell you how much your book *BE YOUR OWN DOCTOR* has meant to me in helping my family become vegetarians. And especially since it has been no risk to health.

My husband and I plan to use some of your ideas when we start our spiritual retreat in Arkansas near Eureka Springs. Perhaps we will meet you before that time."

I am looking forward to reading your other books on nutrition.

"Thanking you so much for sharing your health secrets as well as your beautiful philosophy with the world. Hand in hand, and blessings."   D. F.   Tennessee

BLOOD PRESSURE —

"Even as a child I seemed to have high blood pressure. My face was always flushed, and the least exertion sent my heart pounding. When I married and the children began to fill the house, my real troubles began. My sister suggested I try the wheatgrass therapy. Thanks to my husband's labor, I had three boxes of wheatgrass growing. Two weeks later my doctor said my pressure had fallen "37 points" and the week following 17 more. So the danger is passed and has been for over half a year. I cannot thank you enough."

                                        N. S.   Montana

BOILS —

"My young son Frank had been having a series of boils on his neck. They were both annoying and painful and he was getting discouraged. Some friends said that boils have to "run their course" and he might as well get used to them as there would be twenty-one in all. However, I felt that this was not true, and when I heard about wheatgrass at church, I started Frank raising some in the shade in our backyard. Very soon he was taking two drinks of the juice each day. In addition, I got him to stop drinking cokes and stop eating hamburgers, pies, and other trash a young boy usually eats with his friends. The last boil, number seven, appeared more than five months ago. It was small and did not come to a head."

                                        E. B.   Virginia

"The doctors call it Bright's Disease, but I knew it only as a terrific pain in the back that never seemed to end and kept me bent over. It is supposed to be a kidney that is inflamed and refuses to act normally. I hate to think of the hours I spent in a chair, almost unable to move. Of course, as the doctors say, it comes and goes, but it seemed always awful near. A very thoughtful friend of mine gave me the "Wheatgrass— God's Manna" booklet which I read carefully.

Then the little girl downstairs, God bless her, began raising the wheatgrass for me. The glorious day was about three weeks after I had started when I was able to move downstairs without help and lean over her shoulder in the yard as she was working with the grass."

A. K.   South Carolina

CANCER — BREAST —

"I had a lump on the under part of my left breast for over a year and a half. It was growing slowly but steadily. My doctor and our clinic said it was cancer. They advised an operation before it grew too large. Having read what you had accomplished with cancers through the use of wheatgrass, I got hold of your literature and have been taking the wheatgrass therapy for three months. The lump is now the size of a walnut where previously is was the size of a baseball. Also, it is now soft and there is no pain. My doctor feels I am on my way to recovery without an operation."

E. A.   New York

CONSTIPATION —

"I had been constipated for years and had suffered all the usual accompanying effects—piles, hemorrhoids, blood, etc. I had been in and out of hospitals. I could not even count the clinics on all my fingers and toes which I have visited. However, I am here today, rejuvenated, happy and free as when I was a kid in high school. I have all this to place on your doorstep, Dr. Ann. Prayers and wheatgrass, working together, have really made a new man of this door-to-door salesman. My daily chore has once more become an enjoyment."

H. B.   Tennessee

DIABETES —

"I must tell you about myself. The wheatgrass therapy has made a new man of me. Eleven months ago, I had diabetes; my circulatory system was so bad, my tear glands weren't functioning; my digestive organs were shot. I was spending between sixty and seventy dollars per month on drugs and vitamins and getting worse.

My doctor, a good physician and very dear and old friend, shook his head and said, "There's nothing more I can do." Even though I did not speak of it, I was giving up. Just then as a ray of sun peeps through the clouds, I was given a ray of hope, another chance.

I mentioned my diabetic condition to my neighbor, Mrs. H—— M——. Concerned about me, she told me about the wheatgrass program and how it helped so many of her friends. As she was sprouting wheat to help maintain her family's health, she gave me a box and loaned me a book, *Why Suffer?*

I immediately went to sprouting and put the program into effect.

In two weeks I noticed a drop in my blood sugar; within three weeks, my blood sugar was normal. At this writing, it is "101". Soon after, my other problems showed tremendous improvement. On learning and understanding how the wheatgrass replaces the missing ingredients in my body, because of many years of eating devitalized foods, I adopted the *WHOLE*

WHEAT GRASS PROGRAM —

"A visit to the Hippocrates Health Institute put the finishing touches. The Love, Friendship, and Happiness I found there is for me. Today, I am happy, healthy, and seventy-four years young. I am happiest when I am helping others, which are many."   H. L. B.   Louisiana

EMPHYSEMA —

"My husband has been a victim of emphysema for several years. Lately, he could only take a few steps at a time. Then he would have to stop and gasp for air. I do not believe he would have lived very long if it were not for the wheatgrass. I could only raise enough for one good glassful each day. However, within a month he became a new man. The shortness of breath was gone, and today he helps with everything, lifts, lugs, and works all day."   **P. M.**   Vermont

EYES —

"I am glad to set forth the details of my health improvement while at the Mansion. I feel that it would be wrong to remain silent and not let others know what happened to me. My eyes are back to normal once more and although I am now sixty-nine, I really feel like I am forty-nine. I recall vividly about a year ago I met a man at the Mansion who was over ninety and compared with him I certainly looked and felt like a sick chicken. I never realized then that I could have such a new and wonderful relief from sickness. I am actually able to do more work now than I was able to do many years ago."

"God bless you and your great work."

P. B.   Louisiana

GLAUCOMA —

"As you know, glaucoma, the hardening of the eyeball, is very painful. Doctors can relieve the strain by draining the eyeball but relief is temporary. Since there is no cure, your reports on wheatgrass and cataracts intrigued me. A friend and I worked up a plot of ground for raising wheatgrass. Despite the fact the taste was offensive, I took the mannas twice a day for two weeks and then increased to three as my eyes seemed to improve. I cut my eating the second week to match your diet. Now, at the end of five weeks my condition is so vastly improved I am writing you this to let you know I am definitely on the road to recovery. Glaucoma isn't incurable at all."   **H. B.**   Connecticut

HAIR —

"I received your literature about wheatgrass from friends and I was so impressed that I was determined to see what it might do for me. I had been so depressed, discouraged, languid, and devitalized. I had used no animal products for years. However, I decided to cut my intake of food and begin to grow the wheatgrass. I took a glassful once a day. After about a month on the wheatgrass, I began to notice that my hair was coming thicker and, strange to say, was the color it used to be when I was a girl. This was indeed surprising as I had been getting much gray hair in the past ten years."

H. G.   California

HAND BURNS —

"When Elsie burned her hand badly across three fingers where she had tried to lift the hot iron pot cover, we followed your advice. We placed the fingers under the running cold water from the faucet for five minutes and then covered the burned spots with wet pulp from the wheatgrass, wrapped the hand in a wet face cloth. In five minutes the pain was gone and in twenty minutes, when we removed the bandage, Elsie said she was all right and there was no hurt. It certainly beats butter or baking soda, and it is on our first aid list now."

A. T.   Oklahoma

HEADACHES —

"As a housewife with two small children below school age, headaches can be a real blight. This one, at the lower part of my neck in back, seemed to paralyze me. Every move I made hurt and yet even lying down seemed to give scant relief. I was driven nearly frantic. While medicines seemed to ease the pain, the old trouble would be with me about "period" time each month. My neighbor suggested I try wheatgrass mannas for it, and she brought me some every morning for a while until my plot was ready for harvest. Then, lo and behold, the seizure did not come in May, June, or July."

C. D.   Utah

IN GRATITUDE —

"Dear Dr. Ann: The stay at the Mansion opened my eyes. You are doing wonders to aid folks who wish to help themselves. If I had known the simple Mother Nature's method as you call it, my husband would still be with me. The enclosed check is for your memorial fund in the name of my husband, Harold. This is the one way in which I can really feel that my dear husband is working beside me in this humanitarian endeavor. On my return home, I saw our lawyer and had a generous gift inserted in my will for this most wonderful health idea."   C. I. W.   Florida

LEUKEMIA —

"I have been taking the wheatgrass regularly. I have one box inside as well as two outside the house. It is doing very well. But here is the good news. After all my discouraging trips to the hospital and things continually getting worse, hope at last arrived. Last Friday I had a blood test and my blood count is normal. I don't know how long this will last, but I shall continue taking the wheatgrass regularly, for I have high hopes. According to medical science there is no cure for this disease. My blood count now seems to prove that sombody is mistaken."   J. R.   New York

PARKINSON'S DISEASE —

"I had been a victim of Parkinson's Disease for many years. It first appeared when I fell over backwards involuntarily and was taken to the hospital where the diagnosis was made. When I was released, I believed I was well again. Then, however, the trembling came to my left hand and spread to my right foot. Fortunately my aunt in Washington sent me all your literature. With the aid of a wonderful wife I was able to get the mannas within two weeks time. Now I will have been on the therapy for two full months, next Monday, and all my shakes have gone. It was like being born again. Unbelievable!"
     J. Y.   Tasmania

REDUCING —

"I am doing fine on the wheatgrass mannas. I have six children and they are all taking the drinks. It has become a kitchen ritual you might say. I can see that the children are more alert and energetic. Their father calls them "'Indians". For me it has been a God-send indeed. My weight, when I started, was a pudgy 197 pounds. Within six weeks, without being hungry a single day, I brought my weight down to 165. I will try to keep you informed."

J. N.   Florida

SWOLLEN ANKLES —

"My ankles were swollen out of shape and pained like an ulcerated tooth. I put them under a sunlamp in the evening, but that didn't seem to help. I rubbed them with salves and I had them massaged. Still the swelling would not go. Then I started the wheatgrass as you suggested, two drinks a day and a poultice of the pulp at night. In three nights there was a marked difference. The redness vanished, and the swelling began to go down. The pain disappeared. Within two and a half weeks they were back to normal."

A. O.   New York

TUMORS —

"I am trying to prevent an operation for a fibroid tumor in the uterus. I am following your simple diet. I eat only raw foods and am taking my wheatgrass mannas regularly. I nearly bled to death three months ago. However since I have been taking the wheatgrass, the bleeding has completely stopped. I am 48 years old. The reason I am writing to you now is that when my doctor examined me three days ago, he was surprised. The tumor had been reduced tremendously. He tells me to continue and that an operation will evidently be unnecesary. God bless you."

R. D.   Oklahoma

ULCERS —

"One of the leading players on the Warriors basketball team had been troubled with stomach ulcers for a long time. He had to keep the condition secret. Both his doctor and coach were worried. Through a friend, I got him to test out the wheatgrass on his condition. Within a month everything seemed to heal up. Of course, the physician claimed it was his medicines, the coach was sure that it was the diet of carrot juice he suggested, but I KNOW it was the wheatgrass mannas I supplied him with morning and night."

R. C.   California

UTERINE CANCER —

"I came here because on December 3, 1970, when I went to the Brookline Hospital and had a D & C, which is a scraping of the uterus, I had an unfavorable result. The doctor advised this operation because I had been hemorrhaging about every six weeks. The report came back that I had early cancer of the uterus and the doctor wanted to have the uterus removed.

I decided to come here to the Mansion and wrote my doctor that I would put the surgery off until June because I was going to try another method. He wrote back saying that I probably would not be around in June.

After being at the Mansion for four weeks, I reported to the doctor and had another test, which he was not too happy about taking because he brought out the hospital reports from the Brookline Hospital for Women and that report did say that I had cancer of the uterus. He told me to either follow his advice or change doctors. Then I got the letter afterwards concerning the most recent report which is as follows:

"Dear Mrs. G———: This is to notify you that the cancer smear taken recently at the time of your office visit was reported as normal. This comes as good news. Best wishes as always."   C. T. G.   New Hampshire

THANKS, DR. ANN —

"As I am certain you can tell, I had a wonderfully enjoyable and educational visit with you, your guests, and your staff at 'The Mansion' these past two weeks. I feel highly privileged to have been able to be here with you. And I am looking forward to coming back some day.

I shall tell more and more of my friends about your important work, and I would be indeed pleased if some of them would come to 'The Mansion' as I have to 'learn by doing' and to gain strength and guidance from you and the principles of living you so sincerely advocate.

If this slight, enclosed token can be of service to you in any way in your work, I would be delighted to have you accept it with my most sincere regards.

I found your staff to be friendly, helpful and very delightful to know in every way. They are surely a group of fine people."
                                                                    T. C.

HOW TO GROW
SALAD GREENS AND WHEATGRASS

It is simple and economical to grow salad greens in our homes. The cost of home-grown organic salad greens may be one-tenth of what we pay for commercial salad greens, which have little nutritional value. The harvest comes directly from our own apartment or house garden—where it will have taken little space and required only thirty minutes or so of daily care.

A tray with about one inch of soil will produce up to seven pounds of home-grown greens, which can then be juiced or blended, or used in salads and snacks. (Plastic cafeteria trays are fine, or you can make your own by trimming down the sides of a cardboard box to one inch.) Begin with a mixture of half peat moss, half top soil. Add enough water to moisten the soil, but be careful not to saturate it.

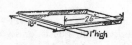

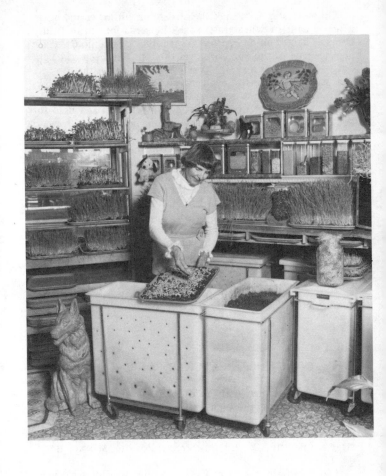

Working in the Hippocrates Health Institute, Dr. Ann Wigmore uses plastic trays as containers in which to grow salad greens.

The next step is to soak the seeds. For sunflower and buckwheat greens or wheatgrass, soak the seeds for ten to twelve hours. Then drain and sprout for another twelve hours. Place another tray of the same size over the top. This keeps the light out and the moisture in. Four days later, remove the top tray and water the greens. Keep them in the light, and water daily, until they are about seven inches high (around the seventh day). Then they can be cut just above soil level and used for salads. Before refrigerating those greens not used right away, remove the hulls.

Buckwheat, radish, or wheat seed for wheatgrass are all planted in the same way. Remember to soak small seeds about five hours, medium seeds about eight hours, and large seeds about twelve hours. Then drain the seeds and let them sprout for another twelve hours, for best results.

The refrigeration of greens or wheatgrass after harvesting will prevent complete deterioration. The juice should be extracted either by chewing or by utilizing a slow-action machine.

Grasses and greens can be grown year-round in any apartment or house.

EXTRACTING THE WHEATGRASS JUICE—

Extract the juice with an ordinary meat grinder or grass juicer. Do not use your blender; the fast-moving blades oxidize the chlorophyll. Not all juicers are suitable for extracting the juice. You can send for juicers by writing to Hippocrates Health Institute, 25 Exeter Street, Boston, Massachusetts, 02116.

The chlorophyll must be used immediately after it has been extracted from the blades of grass if it is to give maximum benefit, for the juice is perishable and starts to deteriorate immediately after extraction. I have tasted much chlorophyll from the drugstores in bottles, capsules, and pills. All of them under such examination, have proved to be dormant and negative with a potency down to almost zero.

STORING THE WHEATGRASS–

Wheatgrass can be stored in the refrigerator immediately after harvesting where it will remain potent and alive for about a week. Wheatgrass may be shipped reasonable distances by mail in a box lined with newspapers. Place the wheatgrass over the paper and cover with additional sheets of wet newspaper. Add a piece of ice wrapped securely in a plastic bag to prevent leakage. You may then ship up to 300 miles. Do not mail on Saturday; the package will probably sit in the post office all weekend.

Visit your local greenhouse and tell them how they can add materially to their income by raising wheatgrass as well as flowers.

BUCKWHEAT GREENS–

Buckwheat has been used by Europeans for centuries. It is also grown in America, but has not yet gained much popularity here. When grown on soil for seven days, buckwheat becomes a superior salad lettuce. Its stems grow to a rich red, while its leaves are dark green.

Buckwhat lettuce is a rich source of rutin, a blood builder, and lecithin, a natural fat and important artery cleanser as well as brain food. When green, it contains an abundance of fresh, rich chlorophyll, as well as vitamins and minerals. It can be used in salads and Green Drinks.

SUNFLOWER SEEDS AND GREENS–

The use of sunflower seeds for sprouting and growing greens is becoming increasingly popular among health-minded families. The sprouts are vitamin-rich meat substitutes—at one-quarter the price of meat—and actually supply more protein than the body can use. Sunflower seeds are a good source of vitamins, especially D and B complex, and of minerals, especially potassium, calcium and iron. When grown for greens or sprouted with alfalfa for seven days, they become a rich source of chlorophyll.

Sunflower sprouts are used to make milks, protein ferments, loaves and sauces, and are good in salads or for snacks. Soaked sunflower seeds in a bag are a great travel companion.

MULCHING AND FERTILIZING YOUR OUTDOOR GARDEN—

Mulch is important for our gardens, not only to help retain moisture in the soil, but also to keep it rich in nutrients for growing organic plants.

Garden material which is usually discarded—grass, weeds, leaves—can be used as mulch. The plants should first be thoroughly watered before the mulch is spread around them. We should then water about once a week, making sure that the water has soaked through the mulch and soil down to the roots. It is suggested that before replanting, we cultivate the mulch into the soil in order to enrich it.

An additional method of enriching the soil is to plant sprouted wheat directly on top of the soil, which is then covered with plastic to ward off the birds. When the sprouts have grown to about seven inches, they are then plowed under. This procedure should be repeated at least three times during the year, and can be carried out on a large tract of farmland or in a small garden patch. In either case, we will achieve organic earth, even though the soil may originally have been chemically fertilized.

HOW TO COMPOST INDOORS—

To compost indoors, box off a portion of your cellar on which to place a layer of earth, then a layer of kitchen scraps (eliminating meat and fish) and any other available organic waste material. Over this goes another layer of earth in which there are a few earthworms; these creatures have a tremendous influence on soil rejuvenation and also aerate the soil. Cover the whole with a plastic sheet. Within a few weeks, the covered material should have decomposed. (When we make this type of compost, we need not have any peat moss.)

Here is another method of composting indoors, especially

for those who do not have a cellar:

Have ready two trash cans. In the end of one of these, drill holes for ventilation and place in it the best soil you can find. In the other, put down a thin layer of this earth and a few earthworms. On top of this layer, place your table scraps, but do not use fruit.

Each day follow this procedure: cover up the day's table scraps with a thin layer of earth from the first can until the second can is filled. Then start another in the same manner; in about two months, you will have healthy earth.

If you are growing greens or wheatgrass, you can put the mats into the can with the table scraps, or cover the scraps with the broken mats.

OTHER VALUABLE USES OF WHEATGRASS

As A Sterilization Property in the Lab —

Dr. Earp-Thomas utilized the chlorophyll for the sterilization of his instruments and for washing his hands when working with various types of bacteria. He found it more effective than boiling water.

For Protection From Radiation —

The United States Army exposed guinea pigs to lethal doses of radiation. The guinea pigs fed chlorophyll-rich vegetables such as cabbage and broccoli had half the mortality rate as those fed a non-chlorophyll diet. Wheatgrass seems to protectively shield against the fall-out poisons when used in the bath and drinking water. Carried in your handbag, it could save your life.

In addition, a bunch of wheatgrass chewed while shopping, taking a walk, etc., seems to neutralize the effects of pollution in the air. Grown in the home, wheatgrass seems to be an excellent air freshener and neutralizes the toxins present in the air.

As a Neutralizer of Dangerous Chemicals in Food and Water —

Dr. Earp-Thomas added a few blades of wheatgrass to floridated water for several minutes. When the grass was removed and the water tested, no fluorine was traceable. Later, an official of the Water Department of New York City tested fluoridated water in which a small sprig of wheatgrass had been swished. He could find no trace of fluorine. Evidently, the presence of wheatgrass in fluoridated water renders the inorganic chemicals harmless. Dr. Earp-Thomas found that an ounce of grass in a gallon of fluoridated water would turn the fluorine into harmless calcium-phosphate-fluoride compounds. Alfalfa seeds will grow in treated water but will merely rot in untreated tap water. One-half ounce of wheatgrass, added each morning to ordinary tap water, softens it and makes it positive. Use in wash water it adds softness to the face and hands. In the bath, it is most soothing. It stops bleeding, eases itching, and helps sores and pimples to heal.

Dr. Earp-Thomas further discovered that fruits and vegetables contaminated by sprays were thoroughly cleansed and the negative food transformed by wash water with a wisp of wheatgrass placed in the water. In pasteurized milk, baby foods, pet foods, etc. wheatgrass changes the toxic orbit of electrons to positive. Wheatgrass placed in the drinking water of pets and cut up over their food helps prevent ailments in your pets.

Vitamins —

Researchers report that every known vitamin has been segregated from the wheatgrass in the amounts and qualities best suited for use in the bodies of human beings and animals.

As a Healing Agent for Burns and Cuts —

Wheatgrass chlorophyll has been found most effective when used on burns and cuts. It seems to lessen the pain and start the healing process immediately. It apparently prevents infection. (See First Aid).

For persons who worry about bad breath, the chewing of small amounts of wheatgrass occasionally during the day seems to correct this problem. For drivers of automobiles, students on the night before exams, or before an evening of entertainment, the chewing of wheatgrass has a tendency to banish sleepiness and to bring on new alertness.

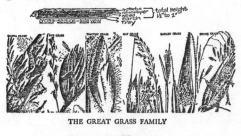

THE GREAT GRASS FAMILY

HOW TO GROW SPROUTS

All seeds, grains, or legumes can be sprouted, although some are tastier than others. Try them all! Seeds can be found in most natural food stores. Be sure that the seeds of grains have not been chemically treated. If they have been chemically treated, the germination rate will drop. Broken or chipped seeds also will not sprout. One ounce of dry seed equals about one cup of mature sprouts.

Basically, care of sprouts means keeping them moist and providing adequate drainage. Your sprouts will mature more quickly in warmer weather, so you would soak seeds less and rinse more frequently to keep them cool. In colder weather, soak seeds longer and rinse less frequently.

EQUIPMENT—

1. A quart- or gallon-sized mason jar or sprout bag.
2. A rubber band or string to secure mesh on bottle or plastic sprouting cover.
3. The seeds or beans you wish to sprout. Make sure the jar has enough room for seeds to expand at least eight times their present size. For example, three tablespoons of alfalfa will fill a quart jar.

SOAKING —

Put seeds in jar and cover with mesh or cheesecloth which you secure with rubber band, or place seeds in sprout bag, or put in bowl. Then fill up jar or bowl about halfway with lukewarm water, preferably filtered water. Seeds are soaked according to their size. Small seeds are soaked for five hours, medium seeds for eight hours, and beans and grains for ten to fifteen hours.

DRAINING—

After the seeds have been soaked, drain off the water. Rinse sprouts twice a day with fresh water, pour off; if using bags, dip whole bag in water and hang up to drain. Now let sprouts rest by tilting jar upside down, at a forty degree angle, making sure that the opening allows air in and is not completely covered up by sprouts. A dish rack is useful for this. Keep out of direct sunlight.

RINSING—

Rinse and drain well two or three times a day for three to seven days. Use cool water. Be sure the sprouts are sufficiently and continually drained, as too much water and too little air will lead to molding and spoilage. The primary purpose of rinsing is to make sure sprouts are kept moist. (Remember to rinse more frequently in hotter, more humid weather.)

HARVESTING OF SPROUTS—

The outside layers of seeds (hulls) are removed in a process called "harvesting" before eating.

Seeds needn't be hulled during the sprouting process.

Alfalfa, radish, red clover, and mung respond well to harvesting.

Fenugreek, sunflower, peas, grains, and lentils don't need harvesting.

To harvest, place sprouts in a bowl or bucket, or in a sink filled with water. The hulls will either rise to the surface or sink to the bottom. Scoop off the hulls from the surface or reach underneath the sprouts to pick them out of the water. Place the sprouts back in a jar and drain off excess water. That's all there is to it!

Alfalfa sprouts need to be set in indirect sunlight after five days, so that they can start manufacturing chlorophyll.

(Sprouts are most tender when young, and they refrigerate well. They will keep fresh several days in a plastic or glass container.)

WHY VEGETARANISM — AND HOW

FERTILE SOIL —

Fertile soil is one of the most valuable commodities in the world today. Upon it depends the health of all human beings and animals. When the soil is really fertile, it is capable of bringing forth food that can give to human beings all the nutrients necessary to keep their bodies and minds in tip-top condition. On the other hand, if the soil is deficient, if it lacks certain elements necessary to feed plants, it will give the world food that is deficient. When this food is eaten by human beings, such food will fail to give elements they need to build strong bodies and healthy minds.

What most farmers today fail to remember is that farming is actually a matter of biology applied within an ecological framework, an individual unit within the highly complex interdependent system of life which the Lord Creator has so wonderfully fashioned. Agriculture has moved away from Mother Nature to become less appreciative of fertile, organic earth. As farming has grown to become a big industry and its methods more and more "scientific", the view of farming has become shortsighted and its goals quantitative instead of qualitative. The answer to agricultural production is not to oppose nature by poisons but to learn how to imitate her own methods.

The cultivation of plants does of itself upset nature's balance, and for this reason it is especially important that we learn to work closely with nature so that we do not further upset that delicate balance. If we are to reach the goal of perfect health or even to have it as an objective, agriculture must be redirected toward an appreciation of the biological interrelationships that exist between every living thing, especially in the soil, and redirected away from the chemical test tube.

Much of the lush, nourishing soil has been ruined through the use of chemical fertilizers. These chemicals have been substituted for normal compost which for generations without number nurtured healthy plants. It is another violation of God's Natural Laws when we deplete the soil and then return only chemical fertilizers, for the use of synthetic chemicals does not return to the soil anything of value. The only way to make land rich is to put back into the land dead and decaying plant matter, just as Nature does on the floor of the forest. And that presupposes that at one time the material had life. The leaf at one time was a living thing. There must be death and decay if there is to be life and growth. This is a natural cycle that no chemist can get around. Fertile soil is full of death and life — dead and decaying organic matter, and life in the form of an intricate community of soil organisms. Man's interference with the perfect balance between the natural processes of growth and decay may be the first great fundamental reason for the disastrous state of health in the "civilized" world today.

The end result of chemical farming is always disease, first in the land itself, then in the plants, and then in the animals and man. Synthetic fertilizers stimulate plant growth and force feed the plants, creating an imbalance and producing a bloated product. Vegetables grow fast and large but they lack many of the essential elements. Their appearance may be tempting, but their quality is low. For instance, Frances Moore Lappe tells me in *Diet for a Small Planet* that in 1940 it was quite common for Kansas wheat to be as much as 17 per cent protein. By 1951, only eleven years later, no Kansas wheat had over 14 per cent protein, most being between 11 and 12 per cent. Mother Nature sends all types of insects to destroy these unhealthy plants. And we "scientifically" and systematically spray these sick products with numberless poisonous chemicals to kill the insects, and then we eat the diseased harvest, plus deadly poisons. The enzyme processes in our bodies which enable man to utilize the nutrients from the foods he eats are affected by even slight traces of chemicals. And if few of us are meeting with sudden death through the daily absorption of small quantities of a variety of poisons, many of us are falling victim to malnutrition and serious diseases through these chemicalized foods.

In the February, 1962, issue of the British magazine *Health for All*, J. E. F. Jenks asked, "How much do we know about the total effects of chemical fertilizers in general? They are commonly supposed to be quite harmless, and certainly no one has suggested that they are directly toxic to plants, animals, or humans, if used in moderation. Yet it is a fairly general experience that plants so treated are more susceptible to pests and disease. . . . The physiological processes involved in plant growth may become very different to . . . a farmer who becomes dependent upon chemical fertilizers, often to the neglect of organic manuring, tends to become dependent on chemical insecticides and fungicides, and so by a series of chain reactions, the possibility of chemical contamination is increased. . . . Little is known about the cumulative toxic effects of chemicals in general on the soil and on vegetation and crops. The consequences of this may be serious."

Steady, cumulative poisoning of the soil is one of the big worries of agriculture in all parts of the world where chemical fertilizers and poison sprays are used. The intricate balance among many kinds of organisms is important for many reasons, and any marked disturbances result in the destruction of this balance, if not in the obliteration of these organisms. When

55

the farmer goes out today to "slay his enemies" with toxious treatments and sprays, he discovers that he has killed his "friends" too.

Although except for the earthworms most of this life in healthy soil is unseen by the naked eye, without this living matter, nothing healthy will grow.

Too little attention is paid by the modern farmer today to the importance of soil organisms and the mutual inter-dependence of these organisms and plant life. A handful of fertile soil contains billions of living microbes which are there for a specific and important purpose. Organisms play a de-cisive role in the initial stages of soil formation. By their bur-rowings and excavations, they construct a system of tunnels of the most varied dimensions, thus water and air can circu-late freely through the soil. They are active in the decomposi-tion of plant animal refuse, returning precious nutrients to the soil. Some organisms penetrate deep into the soil and bring material rich in minerals to the surface where it is more easily available to plant roots.

Charles Darwin stated that the lowly earthworm has a tre-mendous influence on our well being. These little fellows are Nature's aid to soil rejuvenation. They actually till the soil around the roots of the plants. Their burrows form channels which allow plant roots to expand and reach deep into the earth for moisture and minerals. These channels also separate the soil, allowing nitrogen to reach the plant roots and per-mitting the moisture to be absorbed instead of running off as surface water.

Earthworms eat and process their own weight in organic waste, humus and soil every day. They expel the same amount in castings (worm manure) rich in phosphorous, potash, cal-cium, magnesium and nitrogen. All these mineral elements are water-soluble and are immediately useful as plant food. The earthworms is Nature's factory for fertile soil. They can produce tons of needed plant food in each area of land. If they increase normally, these tiny creatures will raise the sur-face of the ground a full two inches in six-and-one-half years' time. They act solely by instinct. They are rarely alarmed. They breathe through their skins and they pair together. A normal colony of worms would number about 50,000 per acre of land and would weigh about 350 pounds. During the year in a moderate climate, these 50,000 worms would yield approximately 35 tons of the best plant food in each acre.

In an article in the Boston Globe, February 9, 1972, Dr. Paul G. Scheurer describes what he believes is an ecologically sound answer to our present wasteful and polluting system of garbage disposal — a worm-powered refuse disposal project. "Earthworms, which could eat their weight in waste every day," says Dr. Scheurer, "could replace incinerators, which are polluting our air and wasting our fuel resources. They'd convert the waste into the finest quality compost." The worms would be put in one end of a long tube, enclosing a slow-moving screw mechanism, along with garbage, leaves, septic tank contents and other biodegradable wastes. In about twenty-four hours' time, the waste and the worms would reach the other end of the tube and the waste would be reduced to superior quality compost, which could be used to enrich the soil and satisfy growing demands for organic food. Any nonbiodegradable waste material remaining would be removed from the tube and the worms would be put back in with fresh waste to begin the cycle again.

The mere presence of earthworms in the soil indicates the absence of chemical fertilizers. Soil which has been chemically fertilized is unsuitable for raising healthful foods. There is a dire lack of organic substances to feed the vast community of life which is in healthy soil because the greatest part of the production is removed from the field, leaving practically no organic matter. Many farmers even burn their cornstalks and other crop residues, which directly kills the soil life. Repeated walking on the soil mechanical working of the soil causes the compression of the top layers which causes a further reduction in soil life population, since rain water is no longer soaked up but for the most part flows off the surface.

In his book *Soil Biology,* Wilhelm Kuhnelt tells us that organic fertilizers act directly on the soil population. Soil organisms react to even slight disturbances and the changes of environment brought about by manure are extreme. Manure is essentially the decomposition of excrement, usually at the violent stages of putrefaction, which excludes nearly every normal soil animal. The selection of resistant organisms that will remain in the soil is narrow, and only in the latter slower stages of decomposition do the usual soil animals reappear. The decay of the animal residues is caused chiefly by bacteria, and by insects, especially beetles, which may be drawn to the area. The putrefactive processes do not lead to real soil formation; their end products either escape in the form of gases or can have a deleterious action on the soil.

Composting avoids this difficulty because the substances are brought to the fields in a condition which they are directly available to soil organisms and plants. Composting on a large scale has been practiced for thousands of years in various regions of the earth. Farmers in America used to grow a winter crop and turn it over in the soil to provide compost throughout the winter. You can convert chemically treated soil into organic soil by growing wheatgrass several times during the summer, allowing it to reach about seven inches in height and then turning it under. Organic farming with Mother Earth will promote the growth of abundant healthy vegetation which will in turn aid the growth and well being of human beings.

One of the most inspirational sights is to see trees, probably hundreds of years old, in their natural surroundings. Through the decades, no fertilizer but their own fallen leaves has nourished them. Nature depends upon compost, humus of leaves, grasses, etc. It actually sickens my heart to see the green leaves being burned and the grass cuttings thrown away in our cities and towns. These green cuttings contain part of the sunshine and are highly fertile. The precious nutrients of the leaves are not utilized as fertilizer and mulch. Instead they are hauled away to dumps at the taxpayer's expense. Leaves hold various valuable elements which the earth needs, such as nitrogen, phosphorous, potash, calcium and magnesium. Hopefully, one day Congress will put a stop to the waste of our natural resources.

The human body when well nourished is capable of expanding physically, mentally and spiritually to limits even beyond expectation. Great inventors like Thomas A. Edison, Nikola Tesla, and other noted humanitarians reached into the unknown for their ideas which turned out so beneficial to the human race. These geniuses were enabled to do this not from study alone, not from hours of concentration of the delving into unheard of combinations in the laboratory. Their bodies were keyed up by the proper nutrition enabling their minds to become extraordinarily alert.

These men found in the vastness of their mentalities the knowledge that nobody had brought to light before. Those thoughts did not originate in the brains of these men. They originated in outer space and the minds of Edison, Tesla, and other geniuses were the mere receiving mediums which took these thoughts, smoothed them out, and presented them to humanity in simple words that all could understand.

Take the discovery of the electric light. Thomas A. Edison found that nothing burned without oxygen and he figured out that if the filament from a sliver of bamboo was placed in a glass bulb from which the air had been excluded, electricity would cause this filament to be heated until it glowed, giving light but not burning. And so the first electric bulbs were equipped with slivers of curled bamboo. Later, this bamboo was replaced by metal which could stand the heat better than anything of vegetable growth.

All great inventions originated in this manner. Ideas come into the brains of healthy individuals. It was G. H. Earp-Thomas, a scientist who was born in New Zealand but made his home in the United States, who conceived the idea that if he could construct an environment of body heat for bacteria, he could build a machine that would be able to digest vegetables and fruit and other organic matter in the same manner that the digestive tubings of the human body carried on this work.

So through years of study and careful breeding of special bacteria, he was enabled to bring forth a metal tank which contained many floors. Into the top of this device, he dumped ordinary garbage with which was mixed the same type of bacteria found in the human body. It entered the top of this device at ordinary temperature and a series of small plows or pushers on each floor gradually worked the material about until it was finally brought to a hole. Here, by gravity, it fell to the floor below where other plows pushed it about until it was ready for further digestion and fell through another hole onto the floor below. There were approximately a dozen floors in this machine, and the bacteria in each floor, acting upon the vegetable matter, raised its temperature to the exact temperature created in the body during digestion by bacteria of the food we eat, or in times of fasting by the fat stored in the body

Dr. Earp-Thomas went further than the mere digestion of food in this machine. He allowed the bacteria more leeway and the temperature inside the bottom of the tank, having risen steadily in the vegetable matter as it progressed from the top toward the bottom of the device, was so warm that steam came from the vents in the sides.

In his letter of December 7, 1960, to me Dr. Earp-Thomas states, referring to the fertilizer the digestor makes with garbage and other forms of organic waste, "that Dr. H. Lunt of the Connecticut Agricultural College and Dr. Vernon Young of the Texas Agricultural Department made official tests and they showed beyond any doubt that the organic fertilizer produces superior results to any other known method in the majority of cases. . . . We have reports from abroad from Professor Andre Birre in Paris of the superior quality crops and from the British equally good."

And in his letter of October 21, 1960, "Our manager asked one of the largest companies in England to investigate the claims that I had made about the fertilizer and about the Digestor. . . Had the reports been unfavorable, it would have been very serious for us but they were not only good but it showed that we had the only system in the world that could make a good compost and the 50 ton Digestor they examined operating had made a profit the first year of $125,325. . . . It does in one day what the fastest other system would take eight days to do at considerable more expense and that the fertilizer made with the Digestor is worth about five times more in plant food values than the compost made by the next best machine system. . . . Reports with pictures show the Organo produced three times greater than compost and was equal or better than chemical fertilizer or various crops tested, and when the plots were examined the tomatoes with the Organo were already producing fruit while the others were just beginning to bloom."

When we feed the soil, it brings forth abundant vegetation. A few years ago, I had a revealing experience when I visited a well known garden which had a world-wide reputation for growing magnificent trees and plants. The plants had been sprayed to keep the bugs away. On the ground, near the roots of the plants, were the bodies of many birds and toads killed by the poisons. Back home I selected a piece of barren earth in our front lawn where no weeds could survive. I composted it regularly with kitchen scraps. Shortly, in this worthless soil, I was producing beautiful flowers, vegetables, and fruit trees, without insecticides. There were no bugs on this vegetation because the plants were healthy.

We should return our composted waste material to the soil. Garbage should be processed to become suitable fertilizer. Nature does not need special fertilizers. In our inside garden, the soil is growing richer and richer from the composted roots and stubble of harvested wheatgrass and other indoor grown greens. It abounds with earthworms, which indicate excellent soil fertility. Folks who visit us remark about the rich greenness of our wheatgrass compared with that which they grow at home. Our indoor grass has been analyzed to contain as much as 40 per cent protein. It can rebuild the body very quickly.

WHY NOT MEAT?

According to the Old Testament, humans began life by eating only fresh fruit and vegetables. The Essenes, an Israelite brotherhood living on the shores of the Dead Sea, had been in existence approximately two hundred years before the birth of Christ. They numbered about 4000 and maintained themselves by agriculture, holding all property in common and sharing each others needs. They were highly religious, did not not believe in the sacrifice of animals, and because they demanded complete cleanliness of the body, dressed always in white. Since they did not believe in harming any of God's Creatures, the Essenes were strictly vegetarian.

Jesus, an Essene, followed the vegetarian way of life throughout his life. When He spoke of meat, He referred to food of a vegetarian nature. The Reverend V. A. Holmes-Gore tells us that the Greek words we loosely translate as "meat" merely mean food or nourishment. Thus Jesus did not say, "Have you any meat?" but "Have you anything to eat?" We ourselves use the word "meat" in a similar way, such as referring to the meat of the papaya. There is no tangible evidence that He ever ate anything but a vegetarian diet of live food, even in the homes of the rich where He was often a guest. Jesus said, "If you eat living food, the same will quicken you, but if you kill your food, the dead food will kill you also."

The Essene children were taught the simple rudiments of faith in God, that they must do unto others as they would have others do unto them, and above all, that work brought results.

A boy of twelve in those times was a mature individual who knew the natural laws of health and had been made to realize that a clear mentality depended upon a clean, vigorous body.

Today, in contrast, many children are held in infancy, shielded from responsibility, and provided for lavishly, in order to escape the hardships which helped build the characters of their parents. Parents smoke while advising their children not to smoke. Wrangling at the table is common, which tends to ruin the digestive organs of the children. It seems more difficult for parents to be self-respecting, uplifting models for their children than it is to allow themselves to degenerate into unthinking, spineless human beings who hopefully advise their children to "do as I say, not as I do". By the time many modern, civilized children reach the age of twelve, they are confused, useless members of society, no more able to face the world than is a helpless kitten.

Parents must "bend the human twig" in the right direction before the age of six or receive their reward later in heartaches, tears and regrets. Wise parents not only discipline their children, but also feed them living food, health giving nourishment, that their bodies will be healthy and their minds may be alert. There is still time to help our growing generation to the path leading to high physical, mental, and spiritual heights, thus forming for humanity a far more peaceful and progressive world. And parents and adults should lead these youngsters spiritually, mentally, and physically in the right direction by example and the blessings will flow from heaven.

Christianity is based upon the ethics of the Golden Rule, and the early disciples of Christ, whose life and teachings were beneficial and humane, were noted to epitomize altruistic love and merciful consideration. How can we better serve God and man than by lessening the sum total of human depravity, both in the present and in future generations? Meat consumption is the chief cause of the intemperance, poverty, crime and vice with which our own land and many other lands are cursed. No reform presently being discussed by our social politicians would produce such permanent and remedial benefits to our community as a return to the living, uncooked foods which God originally designed for man. As we turn from this evil habit, with its far-reaching consequences, we combat drunkenness, cruelty, poverty and sin, and we open our hearts to religious influences. For man's carnality and selfishness are the root causes of evil, and these are fostered by and strengthened very materially by flesh-eating. To remedy the evil, we must remove the cause.

The experience of my good friend, John A. MacDonald, shows the power, the almost unbreakable strength for evil, in improper foods. Some years ago, John owned a pet shop which specialized in the raising of white mice. He sold mice by the thousands all over the world. In his enclosure for the mice, he had placed a large bale of hay. From the dried grass, the mice built a cooperative apartment house. They cut numerous tunnels through it, built hanging gardens, cliff-dwelling pueblos and wonderful balconies on which they raised their young in harmony. It was a happy existence of peace and plenty.

John became concerned about the rising price of grain to feed his mice and was on the lookout for ways to cut costs. A neighbor who ran a rather sizeable boarding house offered to supply him daily with the leftover scraps from her tables. John gladly accepted the opportunity to increase his profits. But when the leftover food was substituted for the grain, a blight seemed to settle over the mice community. Eating the same food that human beings ate changed the complexion of the cooperative establishment. Quarrels broke out and battles raged through the baled-hay corridors. By the end of the week, dead mice littered the floor of the compound; cannibalistic parents ate their young. The weaker mice were slain without any provocation.

Realizing that only disaster loomed ahead, John threw out the scraps of food and went back to grain. And the result was quickly evident. No more mice were found dead or half-eaten. This is not an imaginary story. It is a documented history of facts. And what the "food human beings ate" did to the mice, it is evidently doing today in many disastrous ways to our children and adults in many of our communities.

Here is another incident to demonstrate the havoc of unsuitable food. It is the saga of two sister white cats having litters of kittens in the same bureau drawer one early May. They were both fed a mild, dry cat food mixed with freshly cut up wheatgrass. Harmony reigned in that drawer as the eight kittens used any convenient sprout that was available for the precious milk. The kittens did not know which of the cats was their mother.

Then on May 25, responding to an advertisement on

television, the mother cats were switched from their accustomed food to canned meat with no wheatgrass. The harmonious situation began to disrupt almost immediately. On May 31 the two mother cats were rolling on the floor clawing each other, bringing blood to their white fur. The canned meat was not served that evening, and in its place was the mild cat food with the wheatgrass. This feeding was continued and within a week the two mother cats once again sprawled out peacefully to cooperatively feed the youngsters. The experiment was repeated again to make sure this was the reason for the change in disposition of the mother cats. The results were the same.

Meat eating was never intended to play a part in human nutrition. It is barbaric. Early man, like the anthropoid ape and gorillas of today, had neither fangs nor claws to kill, nor the fleetness of foot to catch animals. Human teeth are not suited to rip flesh. It is difficult to see how man could have been anything but the frugivorous creature that Charles Darwin and Julian Huxley maintain he was. Professor Sir Richard Owen tells us, "The apes and monkeys, whom Man nearly resembles in his dentition, derive their staple food from fruits, grains, the kernels of nuts, and other forms in which the most sapid and nutritious tissues of the vegetable kingdom are elaborated; and the close resemblance between the quadrumanous and the human dentition shows that Man was, from the beginning, adapted to eat the fruit of the trees of the garden." Dr. Josiah Oldfield writes, "Today there is the scientific fact assured —that Man belongs not to the flesh eaters, but to the fruit, vegetable greens, sprouts, and seed eaters.

In a study performed at the Harvard Laboratories of Physiology, Moore showed that a meat diet produces an acceleration of the heart action that is surprising in its magnitude and duration. He found that "after a meal of meat, the increase of the heart rate regularly amounts to a 25% to 50% rise above the fasting level and persists, in experimental subjects, for 15 to 20 hours, a total of many thousands of extra heart beats. It requires the presence of internal poisons to cause the body functions to accelerate in this manner. The evidence of the presence of these poisons is the quickening of the body function."

Carlson Wade, in an article, reports on an expriment conducted by Dr. L. H. Newberg of Ann Arbor University

Dr. Newberg fed large quantities of meat to test animals, which promptly grew to be bigger and more alert than the control group of vegetarian animals. Three months later, however, the meat fed animals contracted kidney damage and died, while the vegetarian animals lived on healthily and happily.

Why is cancer increasing so quickly? It has been noted that uncivilized tribes living on a vegetarian diet are not afflicted with cancer. Yet when these same tribesmen adopt civilized food including meat, eggs and milk, cancer develops. Drs. Humphrey, Bell, Marsden, Roger-Williams, Black, and other cancer specialists have expressed the opinion that flesh eating is one of the chief predisposing causes. Much known information corroborates this opinion, but the chief fact is that flesh food often rots before elimination. . . . and putrefying residue is absorbed into the blood stream from the colon—thus poisoning the whole organism.

After many years of observing and studying the causes of sickness, Dr. Owen S. Parrett became convinced that flesh eating by human beings caused premature aging, fatigue and toxicity. He pointed out that the cells of the body are little units and each must be supplied with proper nourishment to efficiently throw off waste. When something blocks this process, the cells and organs deteriorate and die. If it were possible for each one of us to eliminate the waste from our body cells efficiently, not only could we be healthier in mind and body, but we could materially extend our life span.

The population explosion worries us all because it seems to bode famine and hardship for millions. Hospitals cannot be built fast enough to care for the physically, spiritually and emotionally ailing folks whose problems result from nutritional deficiencies. According to the February, 1972, issue of Prevention Magazine, the production of beef "requires that a cow be fed 10 calories in the form of grain and hay for every calorie that is eventually 'harvested' as meat." In *Diet for a Small Planet*, Frances Moore Lapp tells us that a cow must be fed 21 pounds of protein in order to produce one pound of protein for human consumption. One-half of our harvest acreage is fed to livestock. In a single year, through this consumption, 18 million tons of protein suitable for human consumption directly, becomes inaccessible to man. This is equivalent to 90 per cent of the yearly protein deficit—enough protein to provide 12 grams a day for every person in the world. Yet, in her book Frances Lapp computed that an acre of cereals can produce five times more protein than an acre devoted to meat production; legumes (peas, beans, and lentils) can produce ten times more, and leafy vegetables can produce fifteen times more. Spinach can produce up to 26 times more protein per acre than can beef. Yet one-third to one-half of the continental land surface is used for grazing, while fully one-half of the harvested agricultural land is planted with feed crops.

Although human beings do not generally think of eating grass, this simple plant is actually the basis of much of what we do eat. Dr. G. D. Scarsdeth, director of the research of the American Farm Research Association, states, "Somewhere in the food chain of all people, something green was the starting point." We eat the steak or drink the milk that comes from the cow that eats the grass. The same thought is expressed poetically in the Book of Isaiah: "All flesh is grass, and its beauty is like the flowers of the field."

Today most persons with full stomachs are starving to death. It is not the shortage of food which brings this disaster. It is the overeating of deficient food. Cooked and processed food does not provide the body with sufficient nourishment. Living food provides the foundation on which real health, happiness, and harmony are built. A spark of God is in each human being, animal and plant. This spark should be given every chance to grow naturally to maturity.

The human body represents the greatest work of the Creator. There is nothing more noble and exquisite than the perfectly developed human form. Intricate and delicate in construction, every organ is so perfectly adjusted that it performs its functions with intelligence and with magnificent exactness. Each one of us should understand how and why the various parts of the body function.

We can visualize the human body as a first-class working machine. Nothing man made can match its billions of tiny, interdependent structures known as cells. Each cell is a living organism, just as each of our bodies is a living organism.

We can understand the working of the cells if we visualize each one as a sort of live energy factory. To live, grow and maintain health, cells must receive fuel from the food we eat.

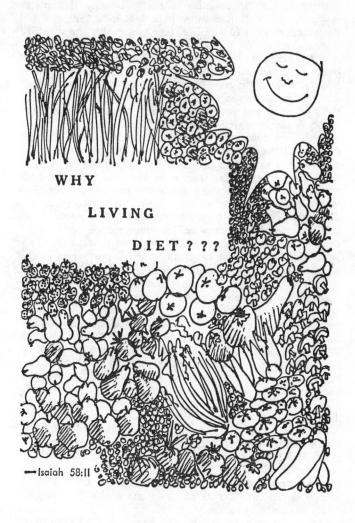

WHY

LIVING

DIET ? ? ?

—Isaiah 58:11

Uncooked food is essential to health because it contains enzymes, one of Natures most important tools. Enzymes are the sparks for the fuel of life. Enzymes enable the digestive organs to digest food efficiently, rendering its nutritional elements, especially the cell-building proteins, available to the body. Air is the fuel for the spark of life. The cells work night and day to keep the body healthy, and they need all the good, fresh air we can supply. An abundance of pure water means youthful cells, and youthful cells bring beauty and alertness. Plenty of sunshine means a healthful life.

Fuel is carried to the cells by the bloodstream. To further understand the importance of enzymes, let us compare the human body to an automobile. If the automobile engine is in first-class running order with abundant gasoline in the tank but no spark to ignite the gasoline, the car will not run. Enzymes, live enzymes, spark the digestive organs to synthesize the nutrients of the food we eat into healthy rich blood.

Blood also brings each cell another needed commodity: oxygen. When air enters the body, it passes through the semi-permeable walls of the lungs into the red corpuscles of the blood and is carried to every part of the body. The cells use oxygen to burn the fuel the blood delivers. This burning supplies the heat for your body by releasing the energy which was stored in live food. The cells discharge their waste material into the colorless liquid that lubricates the tissues, the lymph which transports waste gases back to the lungs where they are exhaled. If cells do not receive proper nourishment, or if insufficient oxygen is brought to them by the blood, they begin to change in character and disease can take root in the body.

Dr. Earp-Thomas ascertained that the lack of enzymes in the digestive system permits toxins to build up in the colon, which in time results in growths, ulcers, tumors and malignant cancer. Most persons are tired because their bodies lack enzymes. The food they eat cannot be utilized constructively but is turned instead into toxins, poisons which lead to sickness. Enzymes apparently, are the key to longevity; they seem to neutralize the basic causes of aging and enable the body to retain its youthful qualities.

Our experiments during the past few years have been most enlightening. I have worked with a man in his late eighties who had retired and was actually dying on his feet. By merely changing his diet to enzyme-rich food, not only did his health problems vanish, but he began to grow younger and could work longer hours without tiring.

The heat of cooking is not the only way to kill food enzymes and nutriments. Excess acidity in the stomach also destroys their effectiveness. The easiest way to add living enzymes of the right type to the digestive tract is to eat ripe fruit, uncooked organically grown vegetables, sprouts and wheatgrass. We need to return to living foods, uncooked foods that have the ability to strengthen our bodies through their electrical impulses, enzymes and nutrients. Cooked and processed food does not provide the body with sufficient nourishment. Cooking denatures the complex structure of the protein molecules and destroys the associated enzymes necessary for their utilization, rendering them less useful or useless.

The average housewife can grow all the food needed to provide her family with the many precious elements missing from processed foodstuffs and chemically grown vegetables. In some climates, outside gardens can be tended the year round. In other locales, most cultivation must be indoor gardening. No outside fertilizer is needed; the earth used can be continuously enriched with the use of vegetable scraps and the disintegrating roots of wheatgrass.

It must be stressed that an abrupt change from cooked, dead, artificial foods to a diet of raw, living vegetables and fruit is very difficult and is not necessarily recommended. In the case of serious illness, it may be necessary. But if you are normally healthy and cannot take time to rest in bed, it is a good idea to use a transitional diet before completely adopting the wheat-live food diet or wheatgrass therapy. For such abrupt change in diet will bring on more severe cleansing reactions and weak or nauseous, which may be impossible at work or at school.

In addition, the transition to living food will be slower for some people than for others. To win this victory, we must forget our likes and dislikes and ideas of the past so far as food is concerned and start anew. To benefit most from this new diet, each individual must study and learn which is best for him. The following routine may help complete the transition to living food.

1. First, cut out sugar, milk products, white bread and bakery products, all carbonated drinks, hamburgers and hot dogs, alcohol, cigarettes, snacks, canned °food, salt and spices, vinegar, coffee and ice cream.

2. Trim the size of your meals and eat compatible combinations. (See Table 1) When you approach total vegetarianism, 80% of your food will be uncooked and only 20% cooked. Add more and more uncooked items until your entire diet consists of living food.

3. Substitute soups and the delicious drinks made in the blender from fruit and seeds for sugar, tea and coffee. Replace cow's milk with wheat or coconut milk. Use bread made from sprouts rather than the usual flour product. For a snack, you can make delicious candy out of dried fruit, fresh coconut, and sunflower seeds.

4. Gradually eliminate meat. Replace meat with cooked sprouts, grains and vegetable loaves. Eat several meatless meals a week. At first you may use fish and the yolks of eggs, but gradually do away with them.

5. To change the diet of a growing child takes patience and perseverance. Young children may have their cheese and sprouted grain bread until they become accustomed to the new foods. All supermarket "goodies" should be discarded and replaced with plenty of fruit in season. Celery and other vegetables should be readily available for snacks. There are many delightful ways to prepare delicious candy.

6. If you have no experience in fasting, skip breakfast. After one month of improved diet, fast on water or fruit one day each week. Initially, fasting is not too important. Improvement in living habits, elimination of the worst foods, and increased consumption of live foods should be your major concern.

7. If you have difficulty changing diets, don't be afraid to cheat. Then strive again to improve your health and diet. After the transition, you will have less and less desire for improper foods. Progressively improve your diet until you eat alkaline foods and small meals.

Good eating habits are essential to the proper digestion of good foods and the efficient, constructive utilization of their nutritional content and other body building elements. Here are some basic requisites to healthy eating:

1. Eat only when hungry.
2. Do not overeat.
3. Do not eat when in pain or emotionally upset.
4. Chew each mouthful at least 20 times.
5. Eat foods at room temperature.
6. Eat juicy foods before concentrated foods.
7. Eat raw foods before cooked foods.
8. If you must snack in between meals, use fruit.

WHEAT —

History shows that wheat has been a prime source of food for human beings and domesticated animals for ages. It is superior in every way to rice and rye and other grains. The utilization of wheat has changed over the centuries, from the use of the berry in the raw state with all its nutrients intact, to the cooking of bolted wheat flour which has had many of the nutrients discarded as unnecessary or troublesome. The health of humanity living upon the denuded remains of this food source has declined tremendously. Our many experiments show that the wheat berry may be utilized to build health.

When bought in bulk, wheat can cost as little as 5c per pound. One pound of dry wheat can be converted into four pounds of grass or two pounds of sprouts or 42 ounces of wheat juice. This juice wil serve a family of three for one week. Wheat berries soaked for cereal or "milk" are excellent food.

In addition to the wheatgrass, our best foods are sprouts, avocado, and greens, such as buckwheat lettuce, sunflower seed greens and radish greens. Greens and sprouts can be grown indoors, summer and winter. From outdoor gardens we can gather nutritious, oxygen rich greens and parsley and dandelion. Dandelion greens are readily available and contain plenty of oxygen, potassium, calcium, sodium, magnesium, phosphate, silicon, sulpher and chlorine. Dandelions are also very rich in Vitamin C. Sesame and sunflower seeds are also of tremendous value. When the sunflower seed is soaked overnight, it can be blended into milk or a handful will enrich your salad. Sunflower seeds can be eaten as is or sauced with the addition of dates for sweetening.

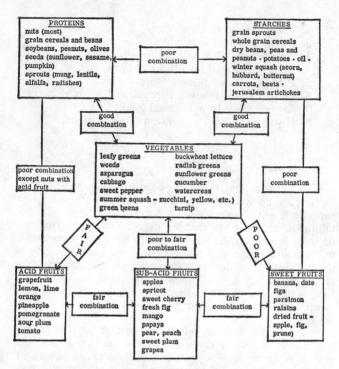

PROTEINS
nuts (most)
grain cereals and beans
soybeans, peanuts, olives
seeds (sunflower, sesame,
pumpkin)
sprouts (mung, lentils,
alfalfa, radishes)

STARCHES
grain sprouts
whole grain cereals
dry beans, peas and
peanuts · potatoes · oil ·
winter squash (acorn,
hubbard, butternut)
carrots, beets ·
jerusalem artichokes

poor combination

good combination

good combination

VEGETABLES
leafy greens   buckwheat lettuce
weeds   radish greens
asparagus   sunflower greens
cabbage   cucumber
sweet pepper   watercress
summer squash - zucchini, yellow, etc.)
green beans   turnip

poor combination except nuts with acid fruit

poor combination

FAIR

poor to fair combination

POOR

ACID FRUITS
grapefruit
lemon, lime
orange
pineapple
pomegranate
sour plum
tomato

SUB-ACID FRUITS
apples
apricot
sweet cherry
fresh fig
mango
papaya
pear, peach
sweet plum
grapes

SWEET FRUITS
banana, date
figs
parsimon
raisins
dried fruit -
apple, fig,
prune)

fair combination

fair combination

Avocados are best combined with acid or sub-acid fruits, or green vegetables. All melons should be eaten alone, not as dessert. Do not mix more than four foods from any one classification. At one meal, do not mix food from more than two classifications.

Undoubtedly there are a host of vitamins which science has not yet discovered which will be receiving close attention as time gradually unfolds their secrets. Unfortunately, many investigators do not realize that all vitamins are rendered impotent by cooking and are at their best only when they are alive and vigorous. Just as amino acids work in combination, so must vitamins, but dead vitamins do not have the ability to work in unison. For example, it is essential that Vitamin A work with Vitamin B to keep the human lungs in good condition, and without this combination, the weakened parts of the lungs and breathing apparatus would take on many ailments and sinus trouble would be rampant.

Vitamin A is also necessary for digestion and to keep the mind clear. Vitamin C must work in harmony with Vitamin K to steady the nerves and bring forth an alert mentality. Vitamin D acts as a guard against the onslaught of infectious disease and helps to stabilize the metabolism. The importance of Vitamin E in solving heart problems is becoming evident, with the knowledge that deficiency in this vitamin will cause deposits of calcium in the blood vessels and also make the body generally arthritic. Vitamin F works in unison with Vitamin E to aid the circulation and keep the skin beautiful through the renewal of skin cells. And Vitamin G is necessary for the maintenance of good eyesight and hearing and to work properly requires the assistance of the other vitamins.

These vitamins must be alive to accomplish their various tasks and to work together to keep the body healthy. Science has not yet learned the importance of classifying these vitamins not only by their different functions but by whether they are dead or alive. Extensive research in the laboratory and the experience of many persons who have tried the wheatgrass therapy and live food diet reveal that wheatgrass juice contains all these essential live elements, and that organically grown, living sprouts and greens are also rich in these vitamins. I frequently chew wheatgrass for enzymes to give me energy, far more energy that any of the so-called "stimulant drinks". Sprouts of various kinds, from grains, seeds and beans are replete with body-building enzymes. A tremendous source of life-giving enzymes comes from the fermentation of wheat that has been soaked in water for several days. This method for obtaining needed enzymes is superior to the use of acidophilus milk for enzymes.

Naturally your main concern will be protein. The children will need extra protein to build their bodies. The amino acid table in the preceding chapter shows that cereals and legumes closely approach man's protein needs. Raw sprouts are an excellent source of protein in its purest form. Since they provide proteins, carbohydrates, vitamins and minerals, sprouts are a remarkably complete food. No chemical fertilizer or insecticide ever touches them. We have found that sprouts may be eaten by nearly anyone with a health problem. The starch and the protein of the sprouts are readily digested with the help of the high quality of enzymes. Research shows such

TABLE 1: COMPOSITION OF SUNFLOWER SEEDS

Carotene .... 0.3 mg
Vitamin A .... 68 I.U.
Thiamine .... 2.2 mg
Riboflavin .... 28 mg
Niacin .... 5.6 mg
Vitamin B-6 .... 1.1 mg
Vitamin B-12 .... 0.4 mcg/gm
Biotin .... 0.67 mg
Choline .... 216 mg
Folic Acid .... 1 mg
Inositol .... 147 mg
Pantothenic Acid .... 2.2 mg
Panthenol .... 3.5 mg
Para Amino-
  Benzoic Acid .... 62 mg
Vitamin D .... 92 USP Units
Vitamin E .... 31 I.U.
Vitamin K .... Trace

AMINO ACIDS:

Arginine 7.2
Histidine 2.1
Lysine 4.4
Tryptophan 1.5
Phenylalanine 4.0
Methionine 3.1
Threonine 3.5
Isoleucine 5.9
Valine 4.7
Leucine 2.2
Aspartic Acid 6.2
Tyrosine 2.3
Glycine 5.7
Alanine 4.9
Serine 3.9
Glutamic Acid 17.7

MINERAL CONTENT:

Calcium .... 57 mg
Cobalt .... 0.64 ppm
Copper .... 20 ppm
Fluorine .... 2.6 ppm
Iodine .... 0.7 mg
Iron .... 6.0 mg
Magnesium .... 347 mg
Manganese .... 25 ppm
Phosphorous .... 860 mg
Potassium .... 630 mg
Sodium .... 0.4 mg
Zinc .... 66.5 ppm

APROXIMATE ANALYSIS:

Moisture 5.27%
Fat 48.44%
Protein 48.00%
Ash 3.64%
Crude Fiber 2.47%
Carbohydrate 12.18%

raw protein to be far superior to animal protein. Their demonstrated Vitamin B Complex content makes them a fine baby food. Vitamin F, a recently discovered substance particularly beneficial to skin and hair, is also plentiful in sprouts. All sprouts contain Vitamins A, B, and C equivalent to that in fruit. Alfalfa sprouts are also rich in Vitamins D, E, G, K, and U. Soybean sprouts are especially high in protein.

And they are delicious, especially when topped with sesame-protein or green sauce, served in a salad. Sprouts are extremely versatile and can be used in salads, cereals, or blended in drinks. Grains such as wheat may be slightly sprouted and eaten as is or blended into malk. There is no limit to the ways in which they can be tastily prepared to yield their nutritional treasure. Their economy, versatility, and their great nutritive value merit a place on any table.

WATERMELON—

The outer layers of the watermelon are the richest in protein, vitamins, and minerals. The Food Chemist, Harvey Lisle, said that if famine ever strikes our country, four of the greatest foods to have on hand would be potatoes, edible weeds, wheat, and watermelon.

The watermelon rind (as I have said) has the richest proteins, vitamins, and minerals. Vitamins A, B, and C are found in the rind, along with their respective enzymes and other elements. If you will examine the rind you will note that underneath the leathery skin is a green rind which merges into the white and then into the pink meat. The green rind contains chlorophyll, which is the ingredient that makes it easily digestible even to people with poor digestion.

Melons aid in the elimination of Uric acid, and are beneficial to the Urinary Tract, Bladder and the Kidneys. The watermelon is especially good for flushing the kidneys, and it will help in dissolving hard deposits that have accumulated because of a faulty diet. The melon is a cooling food and induces gentle perspiration. Melons should be used during hot weather to help prevent heat exhaustion. The "water of life" is found in abundance in watermelons, and they will prove to be the safest means of cleaning the body's waste, while at the same time providing nourishment.

Watermelon is a wonderful aid for the person with an acid condition, as it helps balance the body to becoming more alkaline.

AVOCADO—

A one pound avocado supplies 70 percent of an average adults daily need for vitamin C; a fifth of needed vitamins A, B_1, and B_2; a third of the daily vitamin B_3 requirements; and a generous portion of such vital minerals such as iron, phosphorous and magnesium, as well as being high in quality fat and protein. All this comes at a relatively low cost in calories—about 480 per pound.

The fats are found in forms that are simple, easy to assimilate, and complete. They are cholesterol-free and low in sodium—beneficial factors for a person with circulatory problems. According to Dr. Bruce Pacetti of the Institute of Pediatrics at Cedars of Lebonon Health Care Center in Miami, the avocado is a super-food which can be used to replace meat in the diet. No more than one half to one avocados should be used in a day. They are great in dressings, sauces, with fruits and in salads. Try it in my Cosmic soup recipe.

KELP—

Kelp is the greatest source of organic minerals and trace elements. A quick comparison with other foods especially rich in some of these elements is worthwhile. The iodine content in kelp is several thousand times higher than in milk, iron 72 times higher than in eggs, copper 35 times higher than in eggs, potassium twice as high as almonds. Kelp should be used in small quantities as delicious seasoning.

WEEDS—

For a good supply of necessary body minerals, there is no better source than the ordinary weed. Study a few weeds and learn their nutritional properties. In the library you will find many interesting books on the subject. This God-given vegetation has far more nutritional value than our most highly cultivated garden vegetable. Weeds have to fight to live. They dig out the nutrients in soil that is far from perfect. They live through the efforts they are enabled to make.

The dandelion, uncooked, has more necessary body-building elements than any other weed of its size. It is the most valuable weed, having six times more vitamin A, calcium, phosphorous and iron than garden lettuce. All of the dandelion and its leaves and blossoms may be eaten, but the tender young leaves are the best. Every morning during my stroll, I gather wild lamb quarters. They are the favorite food of my little wooly monkey, Precious. These particular weeds happen to grow in a crack between a stone wall and the cement sidewalk. Another weed that is most worthwhile is ground parsley, and a very popular bit of vegetation is the nasturtium. They make delicious flavoring for salads, and are sort of spicy. A border of nasturtium in your garden is a good move so you will have plenty through the summer and fall. Wheatgrass, of course, is king of them all.

I hope you will consider weeds food, and allow them the opportunity to prove themselves nutritionally. Make weeds a regular part of your diet. Weeds that are unsuitable for food are very bitter and have many thorns. Weeds should be washed thoroughly with wheatgrass in water to neutralize any chemical sprays. They may then be cut into small pieces and mixed with green lettuce. When a salad is made from weeds, sprouts, sunflower seeds and an avocado, it can constitute a complete meal and cost mere pennies. A green sauce or plain olive oil may be used as a dressing. The tender leaves of weeds should be added to the fillings of sandwiches for the children's lunches.

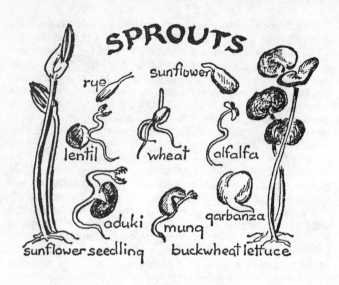

RECIPES

BREAKFAST IDEAS

BARLEY UPRISING —

½ cup water
½ cup hulled barley
½ cup 2-day sprouted sunflower

1 sliced banana
molasses or honey

Soak barley overnight. In the morning, blend with half a cup soak water until smooth. Sweeten with molasses or honey. Pour over banana. Sprinkle sunflower sprouts on top.

Morning Millet —

Queen of the grains, it is the only one that is alkaline and low in protein. Use in unhulled form. Sprout the millet for 3 days and prepare in same manner as wheat cereal. If only hulled millet is available, use it as a warm cereal, otherwise it will have a heavy starchy taste.

Sesame-Date Cereal —

1 cup unhulled sesame seeds   3 or 4 chopped dates
1 cup water

Grind sesame seeds in a nut grinder. Place all ingredients into blender and blend for less than a minute (make sure dates are pitted). For sesame date drink, use 1½ cups water.

Wheat Cereal —

1 cup sprouted wheat seeds   dates (optional)
1 cup water

Blend wheat and water in blender until thick. Add several chopped dates and continue blending until creamy. Or use figs for variety.

FRUIT AND NUT DRINKS

Almond Cow —

1 cup rejuvelac   ¼ cup almonds
1-2 ripe bananas

Pour rejuvelac into blender. Grind almonds and add to rejuvelac while blender is in motion. Gradually add in bananas and for spicy variation, drop in à sprig of mint.

Banana Shake —

1 cup coconut   1 banana   honey   1 cup water

Blend freshly shredded coconut thoroughly with one cup water, add in banana at slow speed and blend slightly. Sweeten with honey. Enjoy!

Coconut Yummy —

After you have enjoyed the fresh coconut milk, crack the nut and take out the "flesh". Break this "flesh" into small pieces, grind to a powder, and place in blender with small amount of water. Or cut up into small pieces and gradually add to water while blender is in motion. Blend until it is changed into a milk-like liquid and sweeten slightly with maple syrup. Yummy!

Dark Banana —

4 pitted dates	1 cup orange juice
1 very ripe banana	

Blend pitted dates with a little water into a fine consistency, At low speed work in orange juice and banana. Delicious.

Dried Fruit Drink —

½ cup raisins	2 cups water
4 dried apricots	

Soak raisins and apricots in water overnight. Drink the liquid for breakfast. Or soak for 10 hours during the day and serve liquid as a delicious fruit drink for evening refreshment. Use the raisins and apricots in a fruit salad or alone.

Energizer —

3 cups water	2 cups orange juice
1 cup honey	2 cups grape juice

Blend together organic juices, water and honey. This is a good "pick-me-up" and energy booster instead of coffee.

Fruit Soup —

2 cups orange juice	½ cup almonds
1 cup diced pineapple	1 banana

Grind almonds in nut grinder and blend all ingredients. Serve with sliced strawberries or other fresh berries.

LEMON SOOTHER —

Take the juice of one lemon, squeeze and strain it and place in one quart of warm water. Sweeten with a little maple syrup, honey or molasses. In India lemons are utilized in most cases of illness and they have proven very effective in giving relief. It is well known that when you feel a cold coming on, a hot lemonade will often halt it.

NUTCOW —

1 cup warm water	orange juice or honey
1 tablespoon nut butter	

Mix nut butter with warm water and sweeten with honey or orange juice.

PAPAYA —

1 papaya	2 oranges

Blend sliced unsweetened American variety papaya with a little water. Sweeten it by blending with 2 oranges.

PINEAPPLE FROTH —

Pineapple is hard to eat and hard to digest. Here is a delicious way to indulge comfortably. Peel pineapple, cut into slices, then chunks. Place in blender with a cup of water and blend for several minutes. To enhance flavor, when blending is almost finished, add 3 or 4 teaspoons maple syrup. A refreshing summer drink. May be chilled by adding ice.

WATERMELON COOLER —

Mash chunks of watermelon with fork and strain. This alkaline drink can be utilized by persons who cannot retain the usual nourishment in their stomachs. Sufferers with too much acidity in their systems find this drink very soothing as well as healing. A watermelon fast has been found very effective when losing weight. It far surpasses citrus fruit for fasting or reducing.

Mineral Water —

To obtain pure water is difficult, you can make mineral water by using your watermelon rine juicing it. This alkaline drink is a tremendous aid to folks who are over-acid.

Another excellent drink for folks who suffer from digestive problems and who are over-acid, is rejuvalac—the overnight soakings of wheat.

FRUIT SALADS AND SAUCES

Almosta Banana —

2 very ripe bananas	1 tablespoon honey
10 almond nuts	1 teaspoon lemon juice

Grind nuts to a fine powder and place in blender with a little bit of water. Blend to a cream and work in bananas at low speed. Add honey and lemon juice and serve over fruit salad.

Citrus Delight —

2 cups tomato	1 cup grapefruit juice
1 dried avocado	

Chop tomatoes and toss with diced avocado. Pour juice over salad and serve.

Fruit Cup —

1 ripe banana	1 pint strawberries
1 apple	1 avocado
1 orange	a little honey

Chop and mix organically grown fruit. Blend a few strawberries and some banana with honey to taste. Pour over salad.

Fruity —

1 ripe pear	1 handful pitted dates
2 golden delicious apples	1 ring pineapple
1 bunch seedless grapes	1 avocado

Slice fruit and toss. Sprinkle with a few ground nuts and a dash of lemon.

HAWAIIAN SAUCE —

1 cup cubed pineapple   ½ cup orange juice
½ apple

Blend pineapple and sliced apple at slow speed. Pour in orange juice and serve over fruit salad.

SWEET SALAD —

2 super ripe bananas   ½ ripe avocado

Slice to desired consistency and serve. Very filling.

MILKS AND VARIETY
BEVERAGES

ALFEE —

Let your alfalfa sprouts grow for a week or more in glass sprouting jars, at all times keeping them exposed to light. After a week or more it will have enough leaves to give you a green drink. If you cannot plant grass, the following method will do very well for wheat or buckwheat. Place a damp cloth on the bottom of a glass dish and sprout the seeds in an area of indirect light for a period of at least one week. This can be a powerful source of green tonic.

ENZYME PROTEIN —

Grind one cup unhulled sesame seeds very finely in a small grinder. Add to rejuvelac and blend to mayonnaise consistency. Sprinkle some kelp in it to taste. Leave this without refrigeration for 2 or 3 days—until it is fermented. This can be used on salads or as is or even with wheatgrass chlorophyll added to it. This is especially for folks who cannot tolerate the chlorophyll alone. This food is easy to digest and can be handled by persons with very difficult digestive problems. Often these sufferers cannot digest protein and generally eat very light food. As a result, they do not get sufficient nutrients to keep up strength and weight and are usually thin.

MELON SEED MILK —

Create nutritious milk from fresh melon seeds—honeydew, cantaloupe, Persian or casaba. After you open your melon, take the seeds and pulp and place in blender with equal amounts of warm water. Blend until it is a "milk" and strain. Add a little maple syrup or honey and serve. Terrific! Remember, do not

REJUVELAC—

Rejuvelac is a fermented drink, but is so nutritious it could be classified as a food. It is made simply by soaking wheat grains in clean water. Plain, or perked up with a little honey and lemon, it makes a very pleasant drink.

It is rich in B, E, and C vitamins, other nutrients, enzymes and it contains lactobacilli, an important aid in digestion.

First, wash the wheat thoroughly until the rinse water is clear. It is important to have organically grown wheat to make this beverage. Soft wheat is best, but if unavailable, hard wheat may be used. It also can be made from day-old sprouted wheat.

Soak one cup of wheat in three cups of water for forty-eight hours. The first batch takes the longest time to ferment. For a continual supply, have two or three crocks at different stages of fermentation.

The second batch is made from the same seed as the first. Without rinsing the seed, add more water to the crock and allow it to soak for only twenty-four hours. It takes less time to ferment since the process has already begun.

Altogether, three batches can be made from the same seed in different stages. The second and third batches need to be soaked for only 24 hours.

Rejuvelac will store in the refrigerator for several days and for as much as a week if honey has been added.

SESAME MILK —

Grind one cup unhulled sesame seeds, mix with 2 cups water and blend into "milk". If blender is unavailable, shake well in a capped jar or use an eggbeater. This milk will not sour but should be used immediately to obtain full benefit.

WHEAT MILK —

    1 cup 2-day wheat sprouts   maple syrup or honey
    1½ cups water   dates or figs

Blend wheat and water for a few minutes. Strain and use pulp
for compost. Sweeten milk with maple syrup or honey. This is
a very nutritious drink and has been recommended for ailing
persons and invalids. For variety, add a little water and blend
again with chopped dates or figs. Or make a treat by adding
carob powder and malt powder. May also be used without
straining as a cereal. If you let it ferment, at least 24 hours, it
will taste like buttermilk and be excellent for digestion.

PARTY SUGGESTIONS

ASPARAGUS BOUQUET —

Place 12 asparagus in a glass dish with radish roses for heads.
Place at center of table and serve with sesame sauce.

CUCUMBER BOUQUET —

Slice one medium sized cucumber lengthwise into 6 pieces
and ½ of another medium sized cucumber into rings. Slice 1
carrot into very thin rings. Place the heads of the cucumber
rings on the lengthwise slices, arranging them in a low glass
dish. In the center of this arrangement, place the carrot rings.

RADISH ROSE —

Using a sharp paring knife, cut the tip of the radish. Leave an
inch or two of the green stem. Make petal shaped slices around
the radish, from top to bottom, from the cut tip to the center.
Place the radishes in ice water and the petals will open.

STUFFED PEPPER —

Choose small red and green bell shaped peppers and fill them
with guagamali. Place them in a beautiful dish of lettuce leaves
and tomato slices.

SALADS

COLE SLAW —

1 cup shredded red cabbage
1 cup shredded green cabbage
⅓ cup grated carrots

small amount onions
small amount dill weeds
juice of a lemon

Toss cabbages and carrots together with a small amount of finely chopped onions and dill weeds. Squeeze in a little lemon juice and serve with soya mayonnaise or sesame sauce or french dressing.

BEET FREAK —

3 medium shredded beets
¼ cup water
¼ cup chopped avocado

2 ounces lime juice
2 tablespoons vegetal
½ teaspoon honey

Blend one cup of shredded beets with other ingredients until creamy. Season to taste. It should taste sour with a sweet tang and salty undertones. Pour over remaining shredded beets. If the sauce has a pronounced beet taste, add more lime juice or vegetal. For variety, add one small carrot to produce pink sauce or replace some honey with lime and pineapple. Use tomato instead of water, or mix very finely diced onions or chives with shredded beets. Or blend in leftover salad for unusual taste and economy. Bon appetit!

CARROT SALAD —

2 cups carrots
¼ cup raisins

1 tablespoon lemon juice
1 teaspoon honey

Add finely shredded carrots to other ingredients, toss and serve.

ALFALFA SALAD —

1 cup water
1 cup fresh pineapple chunks

1 cup alfalfa sprouts
3 tablespoons sesame seed

Blend water and pineapple to consistency of sauce. Pour over alfalfa sprouts. Spread finely ground sesame seeds over salad.

ENZYME SALAD —

2 cups buckwheat lettuce
1 cup favorite sprouts

1 avocado
1 tomato

Cut up lettuce and mix with sprouts in large bowl. Chop avocado and tomato and add to salad. Toss. Sprinkle kelp and oil over salad or try fresh lemon juice.

GREEN GODDESS —

1 part green cabbage
1 part green pepper

1 part spinach
1 part cucumber

Slice spinach and green pepper and mix with shredded green cabbage. Add blended cucumber. Toss with oil. Serve on crisp leaves of lettuce and garnish with parsley.

INDOOR FARM SALAD —

3 cups 6-day alfalfa sprouts
1 cup 4-day radish sprouts
1 cup 6-day buckwheat lettuce
½ cup 3-day mung bean sprouts
½ cup 3-day sprouted fenugreek juice of 3 lemons

½ cup ground sesame seeds
½ cup 2-day chickpea sprouts
⅓ cup cubed avocado
2 tablespoons kelp

Husk the sunflower greens and buckwheat lettuce. Cut up finely and add all ingredients except chickpeas and kelp. Toss salad and season to taste. Use a meat grinder or a blender with the on/off technique to grind chickpeas and place around borders of salad.

SAUERKRAUT–

Sauerkraut is a fermented food that promotes good digestion and furnishes the body with enzymes. It is predigested, cleanses the blood, aids digestion, and helps with elimination. Sauerkraut contains much vitamin C. The cabbage is fermented by bacteria (lactobacillus) that will take up residence in your intestine, produce beneficial lactic acid and synthesize vitamins, especially the B vitamins.

When making sauerkraut, do not use salt. Table salt is inorganic and can remain in the system. Inorganic mineral deposits in the joints can be painful. Even refined sea salt is 99% sodium chloride. A better source of any additional minerals beyond those contained in sprouts, greens and fermented foods is sea vegetables, such as Wakame, Dulse, and Kelp. Sea vegetables are about 18-20% sodium chloride.

Seasonings you might want to use are Caraway and Juniper Berries. Grind one or all of these to a fine powder. Vegetables such as onions, carrots, green pepper, celery, or beets may also be added to ferment in sauerkraut.

EQUIPMENT AND INGREDIENTS–

    2 large heads of cabbage
    5-7 ground Juniper berries
    1 beet
    2-3 ounces Dulse or Wakame
    1 teaspoon Kelp

    (these last two items are optional)

    1 gallon crock or large jar
    1 baseball bat or 40 inch piece of 2x4 board
    1 heavy duty plastic or steel bucket (3-5 gallon capacity)

Grate beet. Shred cabbage, saving 2 or 3 of the better outer leaves. Place the cabbage and beet in a bowl or pail, filling no more than half the container. Pound the cabbage firmly with a bat or board, bruising it until the fiber breaks down and the juice flows out. The more you pound, the better and smoother the sauerkraut will be.

Mix in spices, place mixture in crock and cover completely with outer leaves. Place a plate on top of leaves, and use a brick or heavy stone to weigh it down. Cover crock with a cloth or towel and crock cover, and set it in a warm place (55-75° F). Make sure it is uncovered for 6 to 7 days.

After a week, remove all covers, discard leaves, and skim mold and residue from top. Place sauerkraut in glass jars with tight covers, and refrigerate. Sauerkraut will keep 3-4 weeks.

LITTLECHEW —

1 cup finely grated carrots
1 cup shredded romaine lettuce

1 cup alfalfa sprouts
½ cup finely grated beets
½ avocado

Liquify avocado with a fork, adding water if necessary. Toss salad and pour avocado dressing on top. Enjoy!

MOCK TUNA SALAD —

1 cup favorite sprouts
½ cup diced onions
½ cup diced peppers

½ cup grated carrots
½ grated celery
1½ cups sesame sauce

Mix all vegetables together in large bowl and pour sesame sauce over salad. Serve as is or spread on lettuce leaves. Garnish with avocado and tomato slices.

POTATO SALAD —

2 organic potatoes
½ cup sprouts
½ cup celery

½ lemon
3 tablespoons sunflower seed
vegetable powder

Scrub potatoes and slice very thinly or grate.Squeeze the juice of lemon over potatoes. Add your favorite kind of sprouts and chopped up celery. Sprinkle vegetable powder over this and top with sunflower seeds. For variety add cut up avocado. Be sure to fix the potatoes last as they turn dark.

"SPAGHETTI" —

1 cup 7-day alfalfa sprouts	2 handfuls buckwheat lettuce

Cut off the heads of the buckwheat lettuce and mix alfalfa and buckwheat stems. Around the borders of the serving dish arrange the buckwheat heads. For dressing use sesame sauce or french dressing and top with grated carrots.

SPROUT MUNG —

1 cup mung bean sprouts	1 avocado
1 cup alfalfa sprouts	½ lemon
1 tomato	Kelp to taste

Chop tomato and avocado, add sprouts. Toss and season with lemon juice and kelp. Serves 2.

SPROUT SALAD —

1 cup mung bean sprouts	¼ cup fenugreek sprouts
1 cup alfalfa sprouts	1 cup sunflower greens
1 cup buckwheat lettuce	dulce leaves and lemon to taste

Finely chop buckwheat lettuce and sunflower greens and add to sprouts. Season with chopped dulce and lemon to taste. Toss and serve. Green sauce provides a nice side dish.

SWEET WHEAT SALAD —

½ cup 3-day wheat sprouts	honey
2 tablespoons sesame seeds	seasoning

Grind sesame seeds and add to sprouts. Season to taste with vegetal or kelp or plain seasoning, or with honey. Do not combine honey and vegetal.

TOSSED SPROUTS —

1 cup favorite sprouts
1 zucchini
1 cup water

2 large tomatoes
½ avocado
sauce

Toss diced tomatoes and finely diced avocado and zucchini.
Blend ½ avocado with one cup water and one tomato. Pour
over salad and sprinkle shredded carrots for color.

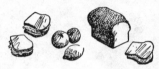

SANDWICH FIXINGS

GUAGAMALI —

2 diced tomatoes
1 medium red pepper
1 ripe avocado

1 lemon
1 tablespoon vegetal
kelp

Using fork, mash avocado to creamy consistency, leaving a few
lumps for texture. Squeeze in juice of one lemon and seasoning to taste. Pour over finely diced tomato and red pepper,
leaving a few pieces of tomato and pepper to be sprinkled on
top of sauce for color. Serve as sandwich spread or as a side
dish to all vegetarian feasts. For variety, optional vegetables
may be added: 1 small diced Spanish onion, freshly minced
chili pepper, chopped cilintro (Mexican parsley), or half a
clove of crushed garlic without pulp, celery, cucumber, lettuce,
raisins or mung bean sprouts.

MOCK TUNA SPREAD —

½ cup unhulled sesame seeds
onions and celery to taste
alfalfa, mung and
lentil sprouts
vegetable powder to taste

1 cup water
1 tablespoon kelp
1 lemon
¼ cup avocado

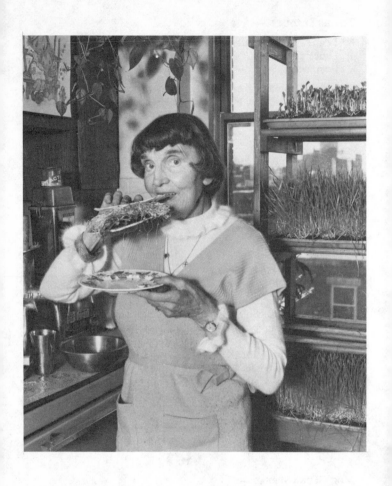

Dr. Ann Wigmore samples some of the special foods that are prepared in the Hippocrates Health Institute kitchen.

Grind sesame seeds with nut grinder. Blend sesame seeds and water at high speed to creamy consistency. Add chopped onions and celery, sprouts, avocado and seasoning to taste and blend. Squeeze in juice of lemon to taste.

SANDWICH SPREAD MIX —

    unhulled sesame seeds   lentil sprouts
    avocado

Mix equal amounts of ground sesame seeds and avocado. Add a handful of sprouted lentils. This spread provides more protein than meat and tastes delightful.

ESSENE BREAD—

    sprouted wheat
    raisins, bananas, apples, onions, or whatever flavoring
    suits your taste

Blend wheat, which has been sprouted for three days, with Rejuvelac—enough to make a mixture of pancake-batter consistency. Flavor the batter with raisins sprinkled on top, bananas, apples, onions, or whatever seasoning or herbs suit your taste. Spread the mixture out one quarter inch thick on a cookie sheet or tray and dry in the sun, food dehydrator, or an oven with the pilot light lit. When completely dry, slice, put in a tight container, and store in the refrigerator. Essene Bread will keep for several weeks.

GRAIN CRISPS—

    grains: rice, millet, barley, oats, rye, and/or wheat
    Rejuvelac
    bananas, carrots, cinnamon, onions, dulse, kelp, Irish moss,
    or the flavoring of your choice

With the exception of rice, all grains (single grains or the desired combination) should be soaked for twelve hours; rice is soaked for twenty-four hours. Next, the grain should be sprouted another twelve hours. Now blend the sprouted grain with Rejuvelac (in a Vita-Mix) to a very thin paste-like consistency— generally one cup of grain to one cup of Rejuvelac.

As you blend, different flavors can be added. For a banana crisp, use two bananas to one cup of grain and one cup of Rejuvelac. For cinnamon crisps, add about two tablespoons of cinnamon. If you want a sweeter flavor, add an herb mixture, and for a vegetable crisp, add onions or other vegetables.

After blending and flavoring, pour the paste onto a cookie sheet or other flat pan; it should be no more than one quarter inch thick. Place pan in the sun, in an oven with the pilot light on, or in a food dehydrator, allowing to dry just until crisp.

SAUCES and SIDE DISHES

CORN SAUCE —

Cut corn from two cobs and blend with one cup of water and strain. Return liquid to blender; feed pulp to your earthworms. Start blender, then add one heaping tablespoon of vegetable powder, one cup diced cabbage. Other vegetables replace cabbage if you wish. Blend thoroughly. Add favorite herbs to this mixture.

COTTAGE CHEESE SAUCE —

1 cup 2-day chick pea sprouts	¼ cup lemon
1 cup water	¼ vegetable powder

Blend chickpeas with water (preferably soak water). Add lemon juice and blend until thick. This tastes much like cottage cheese—delicious!

FLYING SAUCERS —

3 medium cucumbers	½ avocado
Juice of 2 lemons	seasoning

Place a little water in blender and at low speed add sliced cucumbers. Skin and all. (Remove skin if they are not organic). Blend to a fine consistency. Work in avocado and lemon juice and season to taste with vegetal or kelp. Slice up one small cucumber or Italian squash with knife or grinder into thin disks and place at an angle into the cucumber sauce.

TOMATO DRESSING –

2 cups tomato chopped	1 avocado chopped
2 tablespoons lemon juice	1 tablespoon dulce leaves
Italian seasoning to taste	soaked

Place tomatoes at the bottom of the blender. Blend quickly. Add other ingredients. Blend until smooth and serve with salad.

GREEN QUEEN —

1 avocado diced	¼ cup radish sprouts
1 cup chopped celery	¼ cup rejuvelac
1 tablespoon kelp	½ lemon juice

Put all ingredients in blender and blend to desired consistency. Serve over sprouts. For variety, add onion or green pepper or tomato.

GREEN SAUCE —

2 cups favorite greens	½ avocado
1 cup water	vegetal and/or kelp

Pour the water into blender and at slow speed, a little at a time, add in greens. Use two or more varieties that are in season. We have found that Swiss chard and spinach, beet tops and celery, lettuce and celery leaves produce very tasty combinations. For variety, use three mint leaves or juice of half a garlic clove, juice of one lemon, or 1 small onion or 3 scallion leaves. Reduce to a fine consistency, adding more water if sauce is too thick. Add in the avocado and season to taste with kelp and vegetal. Use as sauce for vegetable or sprout salad, or serve as soup.

PURPLE SAUCE —

1 cup beets   juice of 1 lemon
1 cup water   1 avocado
1 tablespoon vegetal

Grate beets and mix with other ingredients. Blend until smooth.
Add 1 cut-up avocado and blend again. Add more lemon juice
or vegetable powder to taste.

SQUASH SAUCE —

2 cups grated butternut squasl   1 lime or lemon
1 cup rejuvelac (or less)   kelp and vegetal

Grate squash and place with rejuvelac in blender. Blend until
creamy and season with juice of lime or lemon and other seasoning to taste.

SUNFLOWER or SESAME (PROTEIN) SAUCE —

½ cup unhulled sunflower   1 cup water
    seeds   1 teaspoon kelp
            or
½ cup unhulled sesame seeds

Finely grind sunflower or sesame seeds in nut grinder. Blend
all ingredients. Some tasty options are 2 tablespoons of oil,
juice of 1 lemon, ½ tablespoon honey, vegetable powder.

FERMENTED SEED CHEESE AND SAUCE—

Protein, when it is cooked, is a very concentrated food,
more taxing to your digestive organs than any other living
food. By "predigesting" your proteins through fermentation,
you give your body these required elements in a readily assimi-
lable form. The proteins are broken into their amino acid components, and are easily absorbed. At the same time, through
the fermentation process, you are taking in enzymes to further
aid your digestion.

BASIC SEED SAUCE—

½ sunflower, ½ sesame, 1 cup Rejuvelac

Seeds are soaked for 5 hours; let sprout about 5 hours. Blend with Rejuvelac and let ferment if you wish (sitting at room temperature) for a few hours. This will keep in the refrigerator for a few days. You can also make milk or cheese out of this sauce, or you can use it as butter on grain crisps. Add some Alfalfa sprouts and you have a delicious, healthy sandwich!

BASIC SEED CHEESE—

1 cup sunflower seeds
1 cup sesame seeds
2 cups Rejuvelac

PREPARATION: Blend and pour into a sprout bag; allow to drip during fermentation. Set out at room temperature for about 8-12 hours. Pour off the whey, then cover and refrigerate. The cheese should keep for at least seven days. Also, you can make seed loaf by adding cut-up vegetables to the cheese.

SOUPS

*Be sure you always add warm water or "milk" to the soups you make.

AVOCADO SOUP —

2 cups wheat milk
1 large avocado

some chives, paprika
other seasoning

Add sliced and blended avocado to wheat milk, then chopped chives and a little paprika. It might need other seasoning. Be sure it tastes good.

BORCH —

2 cups rejuvelac
2 diced beets
1 small green onion chopped

½ cup seed cheese
vegetable powder

Use almond or sunflower cheese. Put ingredients into blender and liquify until finely chopped. Season to taste and serve cool. For sauce, leave out rejuvelac and serve over sprouted salad.

BUFFETT SOUP —

vegetal
hot water
sesame sauce
chopped tomato

favorite sprouts
grated carrots
grated onions
bits of cucumber

Blend vegetal and hot water and sesame sauce. Add vegetables to broth and serve. Or serve vegetables in seperate bowls and let each person select vegetables to add to his individual bowl of broth. Garnish with bits of cucumber.

CORN SOUP —

1 cup fresh corn
1 cup water
½ cup bean sprouts

½ cup uncooked mushrooms
5 sliced water chestnuts

Blend corn cut fresh from the cob with a cup of water, adding bean sprouts, sliced raw mushrooms and water chestnuts. Season with onions or vegetable powder or your favorite seasoning.

COSMIC SOUP—

2 parts greens and sprouts to 1 part vegetables
2 tablespoons seed cheese
2 tablespoons chopped avocado
assorted chopped vegetables to be used as garnish

For one serving of soup, fill a plate to heaping with 2 parts greens and sprouts and 1 part vegetables. Add seed cheese and avocado, and juice mixture in wheatgrass juicer. Top with chopped vegetable, garnish and serve.

Lentil Soup —

1 cup slightly sprouted lentils	½ cup parsley or buckwheat
1 large onion	lettuce
2 cups water	½ teaspoon sweet basil
1 medium uncooked potato	½ cup finely chopped celery
	dulse and kelp to taste

Add to water lentils, celery, slice 1 potato, parsley or lettuce, and sweet basil. Add cut-up dulse and sprinkle kelp to taste. This may be utilized for a full meal or just a "pick-me-up."

Pepper Wheat Soup —

1 cup sprouted wheat	1 red sweet pepper
½ cup water	vegetable seasoning

Blend wheat and water to a fine consistency. Blend in diced pepper and season to taste.

Root Vegetable Soup —

 Finely grind or grate carrots, beets, or your other favorite root vegetables. Add one small diced avocado, vegetable powder, and a little water and blend to desired consistency and taste. Serve as a sauce or soup. Especially good for babies and invalids who have difficulty chewing.

Split Pea Soup —

1 cup green peas	celery, onion
2 cups water	seasoning

Soak green peas overnight. Drain in the morning and refrigerate soak water. Let sprout during the day. Put into blender with a little soak water and mix, adding chopped celery and onion and seasoning to taste (thyme and vegetal very nice).

Add soak water as needed. Be sure to buy fresh, organically grown peas.

3 large cucumbers	juice of 1 lemon
3 large tomatoes	vegetal
1 red sweet pepper	kelp

Blend finely cut-up red pepper with a little water, using slow speed at all times. Add in lemon, followed by sliced cucumbers, cubed tomatoes. Do not liquify; the cucumber and tomato must show. Season with vegetal and kelp. For those who are used to spiced food, which should be abandoned as soon as possible, try using some hot pepper, garlic juice or onion. Before serving, float in cucumber sliced into thin disks, garnish with parsley.

TREATS

3 frozen peeled bananas	½ cup other frozen fruit of choice

Let bananas and fruit freeze to hardness. Blend ingredients, or run them through champion juicer (with blank).

Cut up celery stalks into 3-inch pieces. Stuff with homemade peanut butter. Children love it. Place a little unheated honey over them.

1 cup raisins	½ cup honey
1 cup dates	1 teaspoon cinnamon
1 cup nuts	other seasoning
skins of 2 organic oranges	

Grind up raisins, dates, nuts and orange skins. If cashews are used, soak overnight, and cut up before grinding. Add honey, cinnamon and any other seasoning you may prefer. Do not use any crust. Just place on pie plate and slice.

OPEN SESAME —

Warm one cup of water and put in blender with half a cup of ground-up sesame seeds. Blend at high speed into a malt. Add carob powder and honey to taste.

FREEZER COOKIES –

½ cup chopped or shredded coconut	½ cup ground nuts
	1 banana
½ chopped apple	¼ cup raisins

Blend ingredients with water to a creamy consistency. Spread in pan. Freeze. Slice and serve.

PRECIOUS SPECIAL —

½ cup chopped dates   1 cup apples

Blend dates gradually and thoroughly with 1 cup water. Add diced, peeled apples and blend again. Serve at once.

PRUNEDATE —

5 pitted figs or dates	½ cup water
5 pitted prunes	3 bananas

Soak prunes and dates overnight. Blend pitted and chopped prunes with dates or figs until you achieve an even consistency. Add a quarter cup of hot water and mix. Serve over sliced bananas.

Sesame Coconut Blend —

½ cup coconut
½ cup sesame seeds
½ cup honey

1 cup sprouted wheat
1 cup favorite nuts

Grind sesame seeds and sprouted wheat very fine, mix with freshly ground coconut and honey. Add your favorite nuts chopped very fine and make into a roll. Wrap in waxed paper and place in refrigerator. If sticky, sprinkle coconut over this roll as needed. Slice in one or two-inch pieces.

Cottage Cheese —

Soak one cup cashew nuts overnight and keep the nuts the full next day without adding water. You should find them slightly fermented by evening. If they do not taste like cottage cheese and smell like it, keep them soaking a little longer. Place warm water in your blender and drop in nuts. Blend thoroughly.

SPECIAL PEOPLE AND SPECIAL SITUATIONS

Many who have accepted the live food diet for themselves are unsure about how these foods can be successfully integrated into their children's diet. Others, while usually adhering to the diet, tend to abandon it when special situations—like travel—make the diet seem an unnecessary complication in their plans. The following hints should help you adapt the techniques you are learning to the special people and special situations in your life.

For Children —

The youngsters will find the wheat cereal very satisfying for breakfast with maple syrup or honey or dates for sweetener. Carrots, turnips, beets and all kinds of squashes may be cut into attractive squares for snacks. Corn-on-the-cob and peas should be always within reach. Fresh, organic fruit is the best way to satisfy the child's needs for sweets.

Should you be unaware of the difference between chemically grown vegetables and fruit and those grown in organically fertilized soil, you should take time to compare. Note these three distinguishing features: their color, their taste, and their keeping qualities. You will become convinced that organically grown fruit and vegetables have a better, more penetrating odor or essence because of their live enzyme content, that their taste is more pleasing and arouses the appetite, and that their keeping qualities are far superior.

Teach your child how to make healthful drinks for himself and his friends. For school lunches, substitute seed and sprout fillings for sandwich meat. Equal amounts of ground sesame seed and nut butter (avoid using peanut butter; use almond or sesame butter instead), mixed well with handfuls of sprouts, will produce a delicious sandwich with more protein than any meat filling. Use bread made from sprouts, rather than the usual flour product. Sprouted wheat bread can also be purchased. Sesame milk will supplement the child's diet with protein and calcium. Grind a cup of unhulled sesame seeds and add water, blending into milk. This milk can be sweetened with honey or a soaked dried fruit. The milk will not sour upon standing but should be used quickly to obtain the full benefits.

It is fortunate for future generations that an increasing number of pregnant women realize the necessity of eating living food to adequately nourish the growing fetus. When a child is born healthy, its opportunities are limitless, its capabilities for creation are as wide as the horizon. A healthy body and an alert mind go together. Living food aids greatly in the developing of the total being of the child.

EXPERIMENT —

I would like to share a lesson we learned about Mother Nature's methods through our "kitchen" experiments. We planted a healthy, organic potato on top of some of our composted, organic earth in a tin pan and it sent forth vibrant green shoots so fast that within a few weeks we had to transplant it. As an experiment, we also planted a healthy, organic potato on inorganic, devitalized soil. And it did put forth shoots. But while the potato which "mothered" the first shoots remained solid and healthy, while its offspring took nutrients through its body from the rich soil beneath, the second potato shrivelled, growing darker and more wrinkled day by day, as the shoots drew their nourishment from its body which the devitalized soil beneath could not replenish.

This experiment with Nature in the vegetable kingdom can be compared with what will and indeed does happen when the young mother carrying the unborn child does not take in organic, live foods, to provide the nourishment which her baby needs. The young mother will sicken while the embryo draws needed nutrients from her body which are not replenished by the food she eats. It is most important, therefore, for both mother's and baby's health, to eat organically grown, living, uncooked foods.

HEALTHY BABIES —

Breastfeeding is the best possible way of nourishing your baby, for this is Nature's way. It is easily digestible, convenient and provides the baby with everything its emotional and physical being needs. A mother's milk is a complete food and contains natural antibiotics to protect the baby from illness and disease. A baby being nursed by its mother will make the transition to living food much more easily than a baby accustomed to prepared foods.

At six months, a baby should begin its diet of living food. Abrupt weaning is not a loving way to stop breastfeeding. Part solids and part nursing is a good transitional step. The baby may want to begin with one solid meal a day. The blender is a great help in this change. It may require a full six weeks to make this transition, but blossoming health in a young child is well worth the effort. A baby of six months will gladly eat the food other members of the family are eating if the change is not forced upon it too quickly. Do not expect the child to eat very much. He or she will find, as will the mother, that half the amount of uncooked food nourishes and satisfies far better than the usual cooked meal. If the mother is also using the wheatgrass chlorophyll, it will be easy to add a teaspoon of pure wheatgrass to the baby's food. Sesame milk is rich in protein and calcium and will help build the teeth of growing children.

Get your friends and neighbors interested in bringing up their children the organic healthful way—Mother Nature's way. If you would like further health information on the mother-to-be and on the care and feeding of babies and young children, send for my book *New Age Child Care*.

FOOD FOR TRAVELING —

On every side I hear the comment: "It's all right to talk about living food when you are at home, but when you are away from home it is indeed another story." I demonstrated many times that it is simple to prepare your satisfactory meals while traveling, whether you are in a hotel or in a car. For example, when I was away from my office for six days on a speaking jaunt, I took with me a two-quart bottle with a large mouth.

In it, I put two cups of wheat and filled the jar with water. I left this water in the jar for 24 hours and it constituted my morning drink, which is called rejuvelac. For the next morning, using the same wheat, I refilled the jar with water, forming a drink for the following morning, and so on for six days. In a plastic bag I soaked half a cup of mung beans for 15 hours. Then I poured off the water and washed these beans twice a day. In three days these sprouted beans were ready for eating for several days. Also, having one avocado each day with the mung beans and fruit, such as bananas, oranges, grapefruit, etc., made very satisfying lunches and were easily available for purchase wherever I went.

Of course, I took wheatgrass along. A supply which lasted me six days. This wheatgrass was placed in a container of water which helped me purify all the water I drank and in which I bathed. You can add many other items to your program such as soaked sunflower seeds. Be sure that you fix your mung beans and the rejuvelac before you start your journey. Of course, if you wish you can chew the wheat.

When we move outside the statistics and look logically at

the situation, we find not only a silver lining among the dark clouds but actually a direct road into the Promised Land. This is not wishful thinking. Anyone can test these principles in his own home. At the Mansion, our little family averages ten adults. We have no crank diets. We serve plenty of fruit and live vegetables which contain ample stores of protein, and all of us live a contented, normal life. We grow wheatgrass and sprouts indoors, all year round. During the summer we raise our own organically fertilized vegetables at the Homestead. We shread root vegetables such as beets, carrots, parsnips, and artichokes. Sweet corn on the cob is served uncooked. We drink no liquids with our meals. We have proved conclusively that our program not only provides Mother Nature with the tools she needs to heal degenerated bodies but also that it seems to prevent sickness of all kinds.

The following is a weekly menu to give some idea of the great variety of tasteful meals that can be prepared for the whole family on a live food transitional diet. There are a great many varieties of vegetables of all colors, sizes, shapes and tastes. They can be prepared in many exciting dishes and decorative arrangements to make the dinner table attractive and appetizing. Use different vegetables each night for contrast. And a fruit salad is always a delicious change from the usual lunch or dinner and a light meal for hot summer days. All vegetables and fruits should be soaked first in a wheatgrass solution—just in case—to neutralize any sprays or chemicals that might be present, even organic foods. Unless of course they came right out of the home garden.

MENU FOR THE WEEK

	Breakfast	Lunch	Dinner
Monday:	wheat milk	sprouts and cosmic soup	complete meal salad, protein sauce, sprouts, carrots and asparagus w/grain crisp
Tuesday:	sunflower cereal	sandwich with avo-cado and sprouts Essene bread	complete meal salad, carrot sauce, and sprouts, celery and cucumber
Wednesday:	millet milk	complete meal salad or fruit	complete meal salad and fresh corn on the cob, tomatoes and avo-cado sauce w/Essene bread
Thursday:	wheat cereal	tomato soup and avocado w/ grain crisp	complete meal salad, beets grated mush-rooms
Friday:	sesame cereal	fruit in season	complete meal salad, cosmic soup
Saturday:	apple sauce	corn-sun-flower soup w/grain crisp	complete meal salad and vegetables on hand
Sunday:	prune whip	complete meal salad	sprout salad, cosmic soup

Part III

In Addition
to Diet

THE TRIUNE NATURE OF THE HUMAN BEING

Every human being consists of three components, the physical, the mental, and the spiritual. For the complete organism to work well during its lifetime, all three of these areas must mesh together and complement one another. The scriptures declare that this body is a Holy Temple, an instrument for doing virtuous deeds and for knowing, loving and serving God. We need good health to pray, meditate or perform any service. We need good health to achieve righteousness, wealth, desire and liberation. A life with good health is a blessing indeed.

Our Master, by His example, by His whole life, and by His teachings, showed the path of salvation to mankind, the path of harmony, the path which leads to a simple, natural life. He said, "Those who keep the law will never look upon disease." When our Master said, "Neither heat nor cold nor the bite of serpents can do you harm", he meant that if we live in harmony with the natural forces, nothing can do harm to the body. On nearly every occasion of His teaching, our Master emphasized the law of simplicity as a natural and spiritual law. Again and again in the Gospels we find our teacher stressing the principle of simplicity.

We are masters of everything we possess which is necessary for our growth, but everything which is superfluous becomes the master of us and we become a slave. "Blessed are the poor in spirit; for theirs is the kingdom of heaven." It is a human disease to always try to possess more than is necessary for individual development. If we are all to live simply and naturally, we should be without many of the dangers and complications of contemporary life. There would be an end to violence, for when the earth gives us all the necessities of life, the essentials for our existence, we have no need to exploit others.

God gave to mankind a supreme idea which unfortunately we have not so far succeeded in putting into practice. He showed the human race the way to live and the path to salvation by the humble birth and appearance of His Son and by his life. He showed the human race that just as the sun and earthly life are reborn each year, so likewise must human beings be reborn themselves, to a new life, just as the whole earth is reborn to a new life. We must be reborn not only to a new way of life, but also through our thoughts and through our spirits, for just as cooked, dead foods destroy the harmony of our organism, so do inharmonious and unpleasant thoughts destroy our spirits. And all inharmonies come only if we fail to adapt ourselves to the natural forces. The ancient civilizations recognized that the body is a symphony of vibrations. The organs are the orchestra and the sun, earth, water and air are the energies which give the harmonics to that orchestra, give the body life force.

Good health is that state of equilibrium wherein the mind and all the organs of the body work in harmony and concord, and the person enjoys peace and happiness and performs his or her duties of life with ease and comfort. Good health is that state in which a person jumps, sings, smiles, laughs, whistles, and moves about with joy and ecstacy. A healthy human being has rosy cheeks, shining face, and sparkling eyes. And just as the body is part of the universe, so is mind. At every second, vibrations from the physical universe enter the mind and produce various kinds of influence. The mind of a human being is affected by thoughts and opinions of others, as well. Good health is that condition in which a person has strong nerves and a calm mind and can think, speak and act properly, in harmony with Nature.

When we anticipate a guest, we clean house, make it presentable and attractive. Why, then, should the body, which houses God, be held less attractive, less habitable, less presentable? To feed the body unnatural foods, to feed it too much unnecessary food, is abuse of the body. The more we seek to satisfy desires, to fill this precious vehicle with liquor, cigarette smoke, and unhealthful foods, the further we stray from the purpose and ideal of a balanced life. The body should be loved and always respected and taken care of in order to fulfill the role for which we are created. Good physical health can be achieved and maintained by observing the laws of health and the rules of hygiene, by taking wholesome, light, substantial, easily digestible food, by inhaling pure air, by regular physical exercise, by daily baths, by observing moderation in eating and drinking. Good health can be attained and maintained by prayer, meditation, right conduct, the practice of cheerfulness and relaxation of mind by dwelling the mind on pleasant thoughts.

To seek health in a self-centered manner is to ask for failure. There may be temporary successes but eventually the seeker finds himself right back where he started. Unless our thoughts are loving, we cannot achieve success in any area of life, and this includes the rebuilding and maintenance of good health. To think ill of another, to curse, condemn or to judge is against the natural law and the ideal for which we were created. Though it may be difficult to see God in some people, He is there; they simply have strayed from this realization. Rather than hate or contempt, we should feel compassion and love. We should cultivate an amiable, loving nature and adaptability. By our example, they, too, may begin to understand and know the ideal. Show the way, then, and keep everything in balance. And never forget to say thank you.

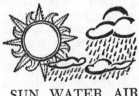

SUN, WATER, AIR
FOOD

We must rediscover an ancient and significant truth about breathing and about life in our bodies if we are to have health.

The human body is a complex living organism composed of billions of tiny, interdependent structures known as cells. Each cell is a living organism, just as each body is a living organism. THESE CELLS ARE ALIVE and every one of the countless number of different types of cells need food. If the cells do not eat, they die. And when the cells die, we die, because we are made up of cells.

AIR —

Oxygen is their life-giving element. It is the cells who breathe, who use the oxygen from the air. The taking of food and giving up of carbon dioxide by the cells is called oxidation. We can picture oxidation as the burning of fuel and throwing off of ashes, which in this case is the gas known as carbon dioxide. Our effort in pulling the air in through the nose and sometimes through the mouth is effected by the cell-effort of the whole body. If we do not work, we are not hungry. The cells likewise are not hungry if they do not work. And the more they work, the more food they need. This process is simple to understand.

The cells eat by ingestion and absorption. When we breathe through the nose, air goes into the sacs known as lungs, in which there are innumerable hairlike little tubes called capillaries. In these tender and soft capillaries, red corpuscles of the blood separate the oxygen from the air by a chemical process. The blood goes through the entire body and supplies food and oxygen to the cells, taking their waste product, carbon dioxide, back to the lungs to be expelled. The blood flows through tubes known by different names according to size or function—arteries, veins, venules, arterioles, and capillaries—each set being successively finer in structure. The blood does not come in direct contact with the cells. The food materials and oxygen ooze out through the sides of the vessels to the lymph which passes through the body along with the blood by the side of miles of blood vessels. It is this slightly salty fluid which gives food and oxygen to the cells.

As soon as the carbon element of the cells has an exchange with the oxygen, the result is carbon dioxide, which is poisonous. Instantly the lymph takes out the carbon dioxide and other refuse from the cells and puts it back into the bloodstream to be brought back by the blood to the lungs to be thrown out. Every minute the blood in the body passes through the hairlike capillaries of the lungs, and for just a second or two, the blood loses the carbon dioxide, the poisonous waste products of the cells, and some moisture. It gains a new supply of oxygen which mixes with the crimson hemoglobin of the red cells in the blood to become oxohemoglobin of scarlet color. And as the scarlet blood rich in oxygen and just leaving the oxygen-filled lungs is going through the great big thick arteries of the body, the red corpuscles are given food and oxygen to the cells and gathering the garbage, the carbon dioxide. When this blood passes through the big veins on its way back to the lungs, this venous blood has become purple with carbon dioxide, the end-product.

Now, in the neck of the individual, there is a reflex spot called the respiratory center from which runs a set of nerves which excite the lungs. When the carbon dioxide becomes too much, it causes acidity in the blood, which triggers the release of an hydrogen-ion to the respiratory center in the neck. This signals the enlarging of the thoracic (or chest) cavity, creating a "void", which causes suction, a pulling in of the air through the nose or mouth, breathing in. From the center of the neck to the walls of the lungs there runs a contradictory set of nerves called vagii, which cause deflation of the chest cavity and thereby we breathe out. There are ducts in the chest cavity where the lymph is sucked in during inhalation and is pushed out during exhalation. As we breathe in, the lymph fluid is coming to the chest cavity, and as we breathe out, the lymph is going along with the blood to the various parts of the body to feed the cell people.

About two pints of air at the most can stay in the lungs all the time, which even by the greatest forced exhalation cannot be thrown out. An individual can take in and out a pint of air at every normal breath, and in the greatest forced breathing can suck in about two more pints, making three pints in all. Therefore, it is five pints of air we play with.

Ease and enjoyment of the Fresh Air should be the keynotes of gentle and deep breathing. If we realize that it is not we who use the oxygen in the breath, but that every cell of the body does, we shall breath differently. In breathing, therefore, we must remember that we are trying to bring the lymph fluid to the chest cavity in inhalation (breathing in) and pushing the lymph fluid out of the chest cavity to other parts of the body in exhalation (breathing out). And that it is the lymph fluid that gives the plasma to the living cells. That the lymph fluid is continually passing things in and out of the blood vessels. That blood and lymph are present everywhere in the body, and that life is the stirring up of Lymph Fluid that it may run in a smooth flow.

We have different planes of action and consciousness. When a person is resting quietly, his breathing is low. Then when he is thinking and still resting, his vague emotional moods quicken his breath. This is the normal plane of life and thought. Now as he gets up and begins to work physically, along with his thoughts, his breath quickens still more. This is the second plane of action and thought. Then we take an extreme case where a person is running or hurrying rapidly through some work with tremendous excitement of his body and thoughts. His breaths become very short and rapid. This is the third, extreme plane of action and thought. It is like an automobile going ninety miles an hour.

When we are running, the cells of the body are eating up oxygen quickly and throwing off more carbon dioxide in quick succession. The carbon dioxide is releasing hydrogen which is going to the neck and exciting the nerves that inflate the chest cavity, causing increased activity of the chest cavity in quick succession. So we have a quick up and down movement of the chest cavity like a bellows and the individual pants. Now one can go at a tremendous speed and yet not hurt himself if the breathing is rhythmic, because in all rhythmic breaths the flow of blood and lymph is always normal, never obstructed by vaso-constriction and tension. If we learn to run in such a way we will not cause any vaso-constriction, the flow of life will go on smoothly.

BREATHING EXERCISES: We shall further explain this breathing mechanism at the end of the story. In the meanwhile, we give here some definite exercises which will benefit us every day. Proper breathing, when it becomes a new habit, will regenerate the cells of the tissues. It will teach the body how to relax properly. It will make us sleep well. It will rejuvenate the whole body and mind by stirring up and rearranging all the necessary ions of the body. Proper breathing will help in digestion and elimination. After a few months of proper breathing, we will find results which will make us grateful to this little book.

Here are three definite exercises recommended to every

man, woman and child. Sit down or stand or lie down straight, so that the spinal cord and head are in a straight line. With infinite slowness and gentleness, and mind, it has got to be with infinite slowness and gentleness, start to take a deep breath. The moment we say "deep breath" we know we will start to hurry. This hurrying will cause vaso-motor constriction and will spoil the whole thing. It will hurt us; it is better not to take the breathing exercises at all than to take a breath with constriction. Therefore, again we say, with infinite slowness and gentleness—because this is the key to the whole situation—start to take a slow, deep breath. Imagine we are holding a tray of ashes before our noses. We must breathe in and out so gently but deeply as not to cause the ashes to be disturbed.

Now we contract the muscular walls of the abdomen, lift the ribs, and expand the chest cavity as we breathe in. Mentally drawing a circle around our waist underneath the navel, from there we feel as though we are pulling up a tree, root and all. Likewise, pull the abdominal cavity and pull the whole body from the waist up, as we take in this breath, enlarging the chest cavity all around. Beware! Do it slowly and gently. Remember the ashes on the tray.

In breathing, lift up the shoulders and send the air to the upper part of the lungs which, through neglect and laziness, becomes the seat of tuberculosis and pneumonia. While we are taking that breath, we must be sure that our neck and face and eyes do not get tight, so while we are breathing in, during the entire breathing-in period, keep on smiling, so that the head and neck and face and eyes will remain completely relaxed. THIS IS THE SECRET OF BREATHING. No constriction is allowed in breathing in. After we have taken in a breath, exhale or send it out just as slowly and gently.

As we walk through the streets all day long, let's practice this exercise every so often so that we form the habit, until the habit becomes our second nature. Our objective should be to make our waist slender, like that of a tiger. If we are fat, this will start to reduce us by increasing the metabolism of the body; if we are slender, this will make us strong. After fifty or sixty such breaths, we will feel completely relaxed. Gradually and gently our whole body chemistry will revitalize itself, bringing about freshness and rejuvenation.

TWO: Let's create this new habit early in the morning before we rise out of bed. If we have to get up at eight o'clock in the morning, wake up at seven o'clock. Open our eyes and lie quiet in bed. Never get up in a hurry. Slowly, very slowly, with infinite slowness, start to yawn. With infinite slowness, turn and twist our body, wring and twist our body, like we would wring a towel. Let's stretch our arms and legs and turn and twist our body from the pelvis to the neck, while keeping relaxed in the neck and head. With every turn and twist, take a soft deep breath.

Inhale and exhale, and turn and twist, and stretch and turn. Make the body as supple as that of a reptile. Take one inch of muscle at a time, mentally, and stretch it and pull it away from the ribs and bones. We must feel it.

WARNING: If we do too much horseback riding the first day, we will have sore muscles and backache. Similarly, if we do too much of this the first day, we will have sore muscles and backache, too. If we are not patient and slow with these exercises, we will have sad results. Therefore, we advise doing this a little at a time, until the body has become supple.

In saying that breath is life, we are not merely becoming poetic. To find out, just exactly what we mean, let's experiment with breath and we will find out the meaning of breath. Suppose we have a cold. We have taken a physic and have further taken some alkaline fruit juices and rest. Still we are not feeling up to the mark. Now, sit by an open window where a current of fresh air is flowing freely. Slowly and gently lifting our heads, we straighten up, sit erect, and begin to take regular and rhythmic, deep, gentle breaths for 5 or 10 minutes. Smile and relax completely as we breathe. We will find, hot or cold, weather outside, that we are beginning to feel warmer and warmer, until we begin to sweat. Stop for an hour or so. Then taken another 5 minutes similar exercise. Wait an hour or two. Once more take the same exercise and we will find the cold is beginning to disappear.

Suppose we get up with an acid condition in our body. We are feeling sluggish. It is probably gloomly or rainy outside. We have no ambition. Everything is going around in our head. We feel heavy and stuffy. Again sit for 10 minutes at a time before the open window and take these exercises. We will find in a short while we are rejuvenated. All heaviness is gone and we feel light as air. The world is beautiful and we are ready to do our work. Breath is a new inspiration.

Suppose the digestive process is out of order, we do not feel hungry, and if we eat, we suffer from gas. Let's try these exercises: Sit before an open window or in the open air and stir up all the abdominal region during the breathing. If we do it twice, thrice during the day, and in bed before going to sleep, we will find a tremendous change occuring in our metabolic process. What, then, does breath do? To understand it, one must understand the philosophy of the human body.

In the cell body there are little bits of radio-gens which are like match sticks, causing the first spark of fire, thus enabling the carbon to be inflamed to burn the oxygen into an active oxygen atom. The nitrogen element in the body, which is like nitrogen in nitro-glycerine in a bomb, must first explode so that the spark of fire will burn the carbon and oxygen together, so that oxidation may take place. This spark of radio-gen, causing the bursting of the nitrogen of the cell, from the psychological standpoint, is called will. Now, when a person smiles and is relaxed, the Will functions better, so that the radio-gens can rapidly cause the bursting out of the cell body. Breathe deeply and gently through every cell of the body, laugh happily, and release the head of all worries and anxieties; and finally, breathe in the blessings of love, hope and immortality that is flowing in the air; thus we will understand the meaning of human breath.

The greatest difficulty the individual finds in learning correct breathing is lack of Will. The average person does not know to what extent they are subject to the slavery of habit. The body would act automatically while the mind wants to go astray in meaningless thoughts of the day. The task is all the more difficult because even educated people of the world pay so little attention to the practice of proper breathing. But we are in a new age where our consciousness is finding itself and reaching for the stars. We know that the new person with this new consciousness will find the right way. It is so easy to enjoy life without constriction. But we make it so hard for ourselves by straining our central nervous system with habitual irregular breath. Psychological reproach of a person for his wild and chaotic thinking and ways of living is of no avail. We must learn the ways of bio-chemistry so that we will be able to control our own consciousness of the body and mind

TWO YARDSTICKS OF BREATHING—Let's catch ourselves at any given moment and see if our head is hot or not. While our head is hot, we will notice our breathing is interrupted. If it is, smile and drop the load of thoughts and anxieties from our heads with the smile. And we will notice, while we are dropping that load, our breath has become normal again. These are the two rules which will enable us to bring health and happiness to our lives. We will become vitally alive persons.

In the bosom of the oxygen atom there is a hidden essence not to be detected by the human eye. This is its very soul. It is nectar. It is this nectar which combines with the essence of the carbon atom of the human cells that expresses itself in the form of electrical sparks of life.

Sit alone by a window before the sunrise in the morning, where a cool, gentle breeze is flowing before and around us. Without stirring even a ray of thought in our brain, breathe softly. We will find an elixir of honeyed nectar in the perfumed air which we are breathing. Do not try to watch it, for it will degrade into solid matter again and the essence will be lost. The blessings of the entire Nature and God are in this air that is free from mercury, dust and other impurities of the day. Beneath the infinite sky above, and the limitless space before us, in the soft twilight of the dawn, as the cool breeze kisses our brow, like the gentle caress of a mother's affectionate gaze, try to breathe gently, very gently, infinitely gently, of this pale air, and we will find the nectar of God in the oxygen. It is this which is the essence of life. It is ever present in the solar universe.

This philosophy with its practical applications shall be taught by members of an expert institute of objective knowledge, the knowledge of Nature, where love for the human being and not money or glory is the objective, shall be given even to children in grammar schools so that we shall have a better human race. Lucky is the person who would understand it and, mutely, in grateful recognition, bow his head to his Maker and say, "Thank you, Lord, for giving me this life every day, every hour, every minute of my existence."

Everywhere we look there is air. There is light. There is sound. There is soft touch. Caress of love. Blessings of Moses, Christ, and all the souls who have blessed Living Creation. Breathe of this life, love, hope, and let us bend our heads in gratitude. For breath is life. And Love—God—should flow freely with every breath.

The sun is the source of all terrestrial life, containing within it everything of which this earth is composed. Without the light and warmth of this celestial body, we could not live upon the earth. The whole planet—the oceans, the earth, every mineral and plant, every animal and human being—is dependent upon Light for its very existence. Throughout all ancient culture, humans have either instinctively, or more or less consciously, recognized that for those who dwell on this planet, the greatest determining force is the sun. And in our universe, all light is an emanation from the sun, the store house of all energies and potencies and the source of all light, warmth and motion on this planet.

The ancient Egyptians, who worshipped the sun as a symbol of the Divine, recognized the power in its amazing properties and radiations to sustain our minds and bodies in perfect health. The earliest literary work known to us in the history of the human race is the Egyptian *Hymn to the Sun,* an apotheosis of the sun which began, "Thou, great source of life, which each day and every year has renewed each of us, animals, plants and man, we await thy return from winter. What would happen if one day thou shouldst not return? Everything would become dead; the earth would die, plants and animals would die, and we ourselves would wait for death, our bodies the victims of the shades of night, for it is thy rays which sustain our life and everything which lives upon the earth." In every ancient people we find the cult of the sun in the form of festival celebrating the renewal of the sun and the earth, and we have a long series of manifestations from philosophies and religions of this ancient pagan adoration of the sun, in hymns, books and traditions, including the masterpiece of St. Francis of Assisi, *Hymn to the Sun.*

Sunshine stimulates the personality and attitude of individuals. A dismal day can sour many people. But let the sunbeams break through the clouds unexpectedly and watch a new burst of energy surge through those around us as they seem to move forward with new strength and vigor. Sunshine speeds up the circulation, helps the lymphatic system and actually stimulates the heart. And the brain becomes more alert. The rays of the sun build Vitamin D in the skin, which must be

119

present if calcium and phosphorous are to be utilized in the circulation of the blood.

This wonderful form of energy which Nature has given us streams forth in Light which enters into the center of each cell, nerve and tissue of our bodies. Each atom and cell is a living thing with its own conscious life and each group of cells is again a conscious living organism. Even a drop of blood is a marvelous world in miniature. These living cells and tiny organisms are in a continual state of flux, forming positive and negative combinations of all kinds, and susceptible to changes in vibration, to the forces operating from both outside and within.

When our bodies are not too depleted and are getting the necessary elements in our food, they have the ability to choose the color they need from the sun. Heliotherapy, an ancient folk medicine, is slowly becoming recognized in contemporary life as a "modern" method for healing and good health. Sunshine healing is one of the oldest known methods of treatment, its history going back to very ancient times, to the days of the early sun worshippers. Hippocrates knew of the benefits of sunshine healing and created "sun parlors" or solariums in which health seekers could enjoy the warmth of the sunshine for healing.

A boundless source of radiant energy can be tapped by taking a brief time to absorb the stimulation of the controlled sunshine. When we are tired, we should take a few moments off to give our bodies a chance to catch up. After lunch especially, sit still in the sunshine, just be still in body and mind, drink in the sunshine's youthful energy. Soon we'll feel the blood rushing to the skin surface, a relaxed tingle, and a ruddy, warm glow to the body. We will feel rested and relaxed. A wonderful feeling will pervade our very beings and a new energy and vitality will surge through us. All this is ours when we take time to let the sunshine energize us with its radiant energy.

Sunlight provides one of the most natural remedies for the nervous person who is filled with anxiety, worry, frustration, and stresses and strains. When these tense people enjoy sunshine, its soothing rays give them what their nerves cry out for —relaxation. As we bask in the warm sunshine, millions of tiny nerve endings absorb the magic ingredients of the solar energy and nourish the nervous system. Sunshine exposure on the golf course or while we walk in the park or down a country road is great fun and a wonderful way to relax. Sunshine acts as a tonic to boost circulation and send a stream of warm oxygen-carrying blood cells to the extremities. The warmth of the sun brings a relaxed tingle and glow to our bodies after the winter cold and indoor confinement.

The ultraviolet rays of the sun help increase the white blood cell count which provides immunity from infection and health restoration through natural means. These little white organisms, as Dr. G. H. Earp-Thomas tells us in his book *Organic Soil*, constitute the defense battalions of the body. This little army of defense, traps and destroys all infectious wastes and any harmful germs that may enter our body. No malignant germ can long survive in a healthy bloodstream: the white corpuscles would tear it to pieces by digestion. Sunshine is needed to stimulate the production of many more of these beneficial organisms, so essential as a self-cleanser.

The rays of the sun vary at different altitudes because of the variations in the moisture and purity of the atmosphere. We should sunbathe in a clear environment, an area that is dry and free from dust and smoke. In cold climates and seasons, we need to sunbathe at midday and when the sun is strongest; in warm seasons and climates, in the middle of the forenoon and afternoon when the rays of the sun have a medium force. Naturally after several seasons of proper diet and a proper way of living, it is possible to exercise and sunbathe at any time and in any amount without danger. Again listen to and comply with the warnings of the organism, our own bodies.

When taking sunbaths, we should always lie with our head away from the sun so the top of the skull is in the shade. Most heliotherapists suggest gradual exposure to acclimate the body to the outdoors. We should begin our sunbathing with a maximum of 10 minutes each day and increase according to our individual capacities. Received in moderation, the rays of the sun will not damage the tender tissue just below the skin. The sun causes special cells in the skin to produce a layer of pigment which protects the skin from too much sun, in essence, the tanning process. Slowly, as the skin becomes tanned, the exposure may be increased. However, we should not let the skin become too suntanned, for it will build a sort of curtain to prevent the healing rays from penetrating deeply into the body.

Sunburns, colds and fatigue are easily avoidable by observing the natural rule of moderation. Like all good things, too much sun is as dangerous as too little. The person who allows the direct rays of the sun to redden and blister the skin is very foolish. The best time for sunning is early morning, up to eleven o'clock, and again after three o'clock in the afternoon in the summer. Overindulgence in sunshine exposure, in addition to blisters and pain, shocks the body. Damage to the digestive and respiratory organs, and to the brain and heart muscles, may occur.

Yet it sometimes happens, when the sun is strong and in the excess enthusiasm and pleasure at the beginning of exposure, precautions are neglected and the skin is severely burnt. Applying freshly juiced wheatgrass chlorophyll, if available, to the burn and blisters will aid greatly the healing process, and cold compresses on affected areas will relieve the body of pain. During the night, put a double damp water compress, freshly prepared, or even better, a poultice of freshly juiced wheatgrass chlorophyll, if available, around the burn and wrap some dry cloths around the compress. Change the compress once or twice in the course of the night. During the day, care must be taken to leave the skin uncovered in shade and exposed to the air. As long as the burn remains painful, or for two or three days until healing is well under way, avoid exposure to the sun.

Color —

All the colors we know come from the sun. Color is the mode of differentiation of the primal light from the central sun according to the different rates of vibration. When the rays are broken down into their various parts, we find the seven primary colors: red, orange, yellow, green, blue, indigo and violet. We evolve from the low gross color of red through the succeeding colors to the highest color violet in the visible spectrum.

White is not a color. White is the combination of all seven primary colors and symbolizes the Divine Spirit, which is positive. Just as the root or plant that cannot catch the sunlight becomes stunted, faded, undeveloped, the individual who is cut off from the White Light of the Spirit becomes ill and undeveloped. Black is not a color either. It is the absence of color and denotes mere negative manifestation. Black produces disease, old age, and death and should never be worn. Both men and women should shun black clothing as if it were the plague.

At the Mansion I have seen color have a marked effect upon the mentality not only of the wearer, but also upon those with whom the wearer comes in contact. I recall one woman who persisted in wearing a black sweater. Whenever she joined a group, she seemed to be accompanied by a depressing cloud. When the others began to remark about how pathetic she seemed to be, I persuaded her to discard the sweater in favor of a brighter one. The effect was absolutely electrical. Almost at once she improved in health and in her attitude to those around her.

This is the age of color in clothes and surroundings. The trend will help to lift humanity to the better things of life. Even men's fashions have turned to color. It is certainly a step in the right direction. Let's replace our white curtains with gay, colored curtains. Select striking towels and wash cloths. See that the bedspreads and chair coverings have life. For those who like color for spot lighting or to accentuate many beautiful appointments in the home, one or more of the color projectors can bring glamor and beautiful tones into our lives. As we add color to our lives for living creatively, the dispositions of those around us will improve very quickly.

It has been proven that color has a definite effect upon the mentality of both animals and human beings. Colors, like other forces and energies, may be either positive or negative in effect either beneficial or harmful, according to circumstances. It is therefore of utmost importance that we should cultivate the right color vibrations in our personal lives and surroundings. The warm colors have stimulating qualities while the cold colors are cooling and refreshing. Colors for the walls and ceilings of the home will vary with the use of each room. The warm colors, such as red, orange, yellow, lemon and scarlet may be used most successfully in the kitchen, dining room and many types of work quarters. They are stimulating and exciting colors. They are most successful in the playroom because they are creative in principle. These colors express joy and warmth of feeling. The cool colors, such as turquoise, blue, indigo, violet and purple, are relaxing and soothing and conducive to sleep. Use these colors in the bedroom, sitting room and den.

In all ancient civilizations and teachings are the records of light and color being employed to heal and restore. The Egyptian priests left manuscripts showing their system of color science a very excellent one. This source of healing has been known and used for centuries and is the most beneficial and natural source of healing. Color healing deals with the finer forces of Nature. Disease is the want of harmony in the system, or in other words, want of color, and the object of color healing is to restore or supply this deficiency. The human organism is a receiving instrument: we receive form the natural forces which live around us and meet in our organism. When not too depleted and getting the necessary elements in our foods, our bodies have the ability to choose the color they need for the sun. The skin breathes and picks up the color it needs and rejects the others. Color is a cosmic power and therefore a vital, stupendous force. It works in and through us, in every nerve, cell, gland and muscle. The whole basis of color healing consists in causing certain molecular reactions in the organs through the medium of the rays. Observations show that people of a certain complexion are predisposed to a definite type of disease and the practised eye of the healer can detect at once the class of disease to which a man is liable.

Red is the first visible color in the spectrum. Although the color red is low in vibrations, it is uplifting as it stimulates vitality and promotes quick energy. Red stimulates the senses such as seeing, hearing, smelling and feeling, etc. It is the color of courage or aggression; it can be irritating or exciting. The effect of red on a bull is well known.

Red is the warmest of all colors. Red is heating, vitalizing, a stimulating vibration and blood healer, and warms the entire body. It is very effective in cases of physical debility, exhaustion, depletion and bad circulation. It is excellent in blood-deficiency diseases, but should be used with caution. As a general rule, red should be used where there is a lack of vitality, emaciation, poor circulation, depression, cold inflammation, paralysis. It helps to clean out mucous and waste from the body. Experiments have shown that plants grown under red glass shoot up four times more quickly than in ordinary sunlight. The reason for this is that red is the "life ray".

Pink is the combination of color red, the warm vital color

of passion, and white, which symbolizes the Divine Spirit. Pink is therefore the color that would encourage affections, to raise the love vibrations in everything.

Orange, a mixture of red and yellow, is a color which helps recharge the body with electrical energy. For loss of vitality and listlessness, the life-giving orange ray permeates the whole being, rejuvenating every atom and particle, filling it with vitality and the joy of life. Orange is a warm, positive, and stimulating color, influencing primarily the vital processes of assimilation and circulation. Essential for health and vitality, it regulates the intake of food and is based on the spleen. Orange helps to cause vomiting when food is not being digested. The orange color stimulates and builds the lungs, activates the thyroid and mammillary glands. Orange is powerful in colds, sluggish or chronic conditions, relieves gas, convulsions and cramps throughout the digestive system, including hiccups.

Yellow represents spiritual intelligence and wisdom and influences the higher mind and soul. Yellow is a positive magnetic vibration which is inspiring and stimulating, with a tonic effect on the nerves. Clear golden yellow is one of the most powerful forces against depression and limitations of every kind. Yellow activates all body functions, except the spleen, increases appetite and aids in the assimilation of proper food for better nutrition. It stimulates the heart for better circulation, the liver and gall bladder, helps in stimulating eyes and ears, and helps build nerves and muscles and activates them where other systems fail. Infantile paralysis responds rapidly to the irradiation of yellow. Yellow, because of its sodium principle, is used most successfully in cases of ulcers to build the stomach, and in loosening calcium and lime deposits. Before these chronic conditions can be eliminated from the body, they must be loosened and dissolved. Lemon is most effective.

The green ray is a vibration of harmony and balance, a relaxing and comfortable color. It is truly Nature's child. Nature radiates this color perpetually; it is soothing and sympathetic and does not excite, inflame or irritate. It is Nature's master tonic, the restorer of tired nerves and the giver of energy. When I have disturbing conditions around me, I make it a practice to wear green. It seems to sooth the nerves of others and keeps my own mentality in check.

Green is of fundamental importance to the nervous system. In the city, our paths are paved with cement, a gray lifeless depressing color. We are surrounded by manmade cement and there is almost a complete absence of Mother Nature's green, which is soothing and calming. And as a result of the unnautral environment of the city, there are thousands of people who are irritable and depressed, troubled with nervous disorders of all degrees and kinds. Everyone of these people can be greatly helped. The blue of the sky and the green of the vegetation deserve full credit for resting the nervous system. It was Elbert Hubbard who said, "If insane persons could be released under the blue dome of heaven with a carpet of green grass under their bare feet, limitless recoveries would be possible."

Green is the master color and represents the chlorophyll or cleansing principle. It dissolves blood clots and affects and stimulates the master pituitary gland for better control of other glands and organs throughout the body. Green is the basic color for all disorders, either chronic or acute. The nitrogen or protein principle of the green builds the muscles, tissues and cells. Blue and green rays act as sedatives and relieve excitement and inflammation. The light shades of blue and green are used in hospitals and have a healing characteristic that helps people get well.

Turquoise is very cooling and relaxing and is a depressant for an over-active and over-stimulated brain. Turquoise gives fast relief from various kinds of irritations and itching, fatigue, poisons, insomnia, and is especially soothing for headaches and many kinds of extreme pressure or swelling conditions. Turquoise gives immediate relief and correction from sunburn, hot liquid burns and severe skin injuries. Some of the most severe destruction of the skin has responded and healed rapidly without even leaving a scar.

SCARLET speeds the heart action and raises blood pressure, thus increasing circulation, and gives immediate relief to asthma and sinus sufferers. It stimulates emotions and sex desires and relieves menstrual pains. Scarlet may be used whenever lemon is indicated to give relief from congestion.

PURPLE gives similar relief from pain and suffering as narcotics give, without the harmful side effects. It lowers blood pressure to give relief from many headaches and pressure pains, such as toothache. Purple gives relief from fever, reduces sex desires and over-emotional disorders. Due to its hypnotic effect, one finds restful and relaxed sleep.

MAGENTA is similar to scarlet and purple, but works

more slowly, and as with green can be used for all disorders regardless of their names. Magenta gives all kinds of changes for heart conditions regardless of name. Nothing can give relief to the heart with such rapidity and accuracy as does magenta. Magenta balances the emotions, giving relief to all phases of these disorders and inharmonies.

INDIGO influences the central part of the head, exercising dominion over the eye, ear and nose, and depressing the over-active thyroid. It is of great value in the treatment of respiratory disease, for better and freer breathing, and gives immediate relief from nosebleed and internal bleeding. Indigo has the effect of a sedative and gives relief from swellings and extreme and acute pain. Acting as an astringent, indigo tightens and tones muscles, nerves and skin.

Indigo and violet are considered to be more spiritual than other colors and are high in vibration. Indigo presides over the higher phenomena of the soul, sensitivity, spiritual perception and intuitive faculties. Indigo has a powerful influence on the mental and nervous organism, can expel the negative elements in the consciousness, and when rightly understood and applied, is capable of building up and inducing the higher, positive elements. Indigo is the cosmic ray of inner knowledge and wisdom. This ray produces a receptivity of mind which is most helpful to students of all classes and especially in psychic and spiritual studies.

One of the best ways of absorbing color is the judicious use of vegetables, fruits and liquids that have been suncharged. Plants are governed by the same natural law as human beings and have the ability to pick up just the color and elements they need, if all are present in the soil and air where they grow. Fruits and vegetables grown organically in the ground are the direct result of the sun's radiations. When we eat any kind of food, we are actually eating color from the sun. The chemicals and minerals are there because of the action of the color in the sun's rays. Of course, the minerals have to be in the soil and air or the colors could not make the plant grow. The guiding principle in diet should be to eat the finer kinds of foods as much as possible, in preference to the coarser foods, and to seek those foods that contain most of the cosmic solar energy.

Chlorophyll is the green coloring matter of the plant and corresponds with hemoglobin, the red pigment of the blood.

Without chlorophyll there can be no vegetable life, as without hemoglobin there can be no human or animal life. The best form of protein is always obtained from living green foods from the vegetable and seed sources. Plenty of sprouts and greens should be included in the diet.

WATER —

The spirit of God is upon the surface of the waters. The ancients were familiar with the knowledge that rain water is distilled from the oceans and rivers of the world by the heat and power of the sun. Sunlight is the world's greatest purifier and healer, and these great powers are to be found in the waters of the sun, the showers of gentle rain that fall upon all creation, and in the clear mountain streams which, flowing over rocks on their way to the sea, deposit their earthly particles and absorb oxygen and sunlight from the atmosphere. The innate powers of nourishment and self purification in all rain and surface waters clearly show Nature's intentions and plan for the life upon this earth. Hippocrates said that "All things are composed of two different but complementary elements—fire (sunlight) and water. The power of fire (sunlight) is to cause motion (energy) and that of water to nourish." Water is the life-giving element of all creation, without which there would be nothing but wastelands and deserts. Our bodies consist of more water than any other element. Water is more important to our bodies than food, for without water a human being would die in a matter of days.

In all great and ancient civilizations, the bathing of the body and its internal and external purification played a predominant role. Alexandria in its zenith under the Ptolemies had four thousand public baths when the population was a quarter of a million. The ancient Greeks knew all about oxygen in surface water and the bathing of the body became a medical science. The fountains of Greece were guarded with great care. One can scarcely think of the Romans without picturing their magnificent baths and the massive aqueducts that conveyed the purest surface sun-water to them.

Hippocrates, the greatest physician of the "golden age", when humans reached the height of physical perfection and clear thinking, postulated that sunlight in water was the basis of the health of human beings. Hydropathy, a Greek word meaning "sunwater therapy", was the foundation of all healing in ancient Greece and other ancient civilizations of the goldren age of mankind, the age of truth, beauty, and love of nature, the age in which the greatest philosophers and physicians healed the sick with fresh air, sun-water, exercise and diet, rest, massage and surgery when necessary. History tells us that Charmis, a physician of Marseilles in ancient Gaul, had only one treatment for all diseases, a cold bath. Yet he charged fabulous sums for just diagnosing the ailment. The Turkish baths, the hot baths and steam baths of the Russians, who roll in the snow after them, and the steam baths of the Scandinavian countries, are older than their history.

In ancient times in America, Indians travelled long distances to hot springs and healing waters. In a book *The Water Cure,* written in 1852 by six medical men, Dr. Shaw relates that upon attempting to minister to Indians in a nearby camp, sick with smallpox, in spite of the treatments, powders and skills used according to the rules laid down in their medical books, a number that they treated died. Some of these sick Indians, however, plunged headforemost into a neighboring creek of cold water, in some instances at the height of the fever. To the astonishment of the doctors, their skin was less pitted and they came up strong and well and every one of them that had plunged into the cold water recovered.

Hoffman, the famous German doctor, says that if there existed anything in the world that could be called a panacea, it is pure water. Water is the grand purifier of the innumerable canals and passages of the human being's complex machinery. It serves to dilute and dissolve the solid waste matter of the alimentary canal, and it acts generally as a cleanser to remove from the body its waste and deleterious or diseased particles. Water is also the vehicle for carrying the nutrient principles into all parts of the organism.

Dr. John Balbirnic, British hydropathic surgeon of the last century, used warm water—the purest in the Highlands—in his treatments which were mild like Hippocrates. He wrote at least eight books dealing with both actue and chronic disease. He discovered than consumption, like many other diseases, was caused by lack of oxygen in the bloodstream and could be relieved and eliminated by use of oxygenated water as well as fresh air.

Germany has long recognized the curative elements of water. Just prior to the present century, three German doctors brought to this country what is known as the "Father Kneipp Water Cure", a method of healing brought into being by a German Catholic priest to give to the poor of his parish a means of helping themselves inexpensively. This healing method centered about the use of water for baths, flushes, sprays, etc., both hot and cold. Father Kneipp proved the efficacy of this discovery by healing the ailing of nearly every known disease. He found that hot and cold applications of water to a sore enabled Nature to mend the trouble in half the time usually required. Walking on dewy grass opened up the large pores in the feet allowing the waste from the body to drain out. The rich emanations from the earth gave new strength and stamina to the cells. The drinking of pure water at body temperature, he learned, was Nature's great healing agent because it lubricated the cells of the human body. Hot, moist heat relieved abdominal pains. Large quantities of warm water flushed out the digestive tubings and toned up the sluggish colon. Warm baths relaxed tensions and eased muscle strains. There was nothing to equal cooling water for burns.

Dr. Joseph M. Price suggests that there is a definite correlation between the introduction and widespread use of chlorine in our drinking water and the origin and increasing incidence of heart disease. Both chlorine and fluorine inhibit the action of the health-giving organisms—enzymes—which must be present for the digestion of food. Dr. Ludwik Gross, cancer researcher, describes fluorine as "an insidious poison, toxic and cumulative in its effects" and the 24th edition of *U.S. Dispensary* described it as a "violent poison to all living tissue." Yet, our scientists, ignoring the real cause of tooth decay, offer this poisonous substance as a spectacular, quick "cure" for tooth decay, and their experiments are not designed to find out whether fluoridation is beneficial or harmful to the well being of the entire person, but to sell their Idea. Dr. Frederick B. Exner, Fellow of the American College of Radiology, University of Washington, says that while "It is true that there are places where there is more fluoride and less tooth decay, there are also places where the reverse is true. We aren't told about the latter."

A country which cared for the health of its people would supply its communities with pure drinking water. The French who consider the quality of water of more importance than we do, do not chlorinate it. Their government advertises the spas and healing waters of the whole country. They have better teeth than we have as a nation and quicker brains if we judge by traffic in Paris which goes twice as fast while street accidents are a fraction of ours.

The evening sitz bath, sitting in a tub containing enough comfortably warm water to cover the lower part or the abdomen, is very beneficial in drawing the blood away from the brain, relaxing us from the tensions and stresses of the day, and stimulating a healthy appetite. If we lie back so that only our head is above water, we soak up relaxing warmth and energy. The length of such a bath should be about five minutes.

When I was still a young girl, I went to live and work on a farm some miles from the home of my grandmother, seeking to earn my fare to America. And all during the four years I spent as part of that wonderful family of five women, our weekly ritual of the Saturday Night Bath was as regular as the coming of Saturday. Winter, summer, spring and fall, in heat or blizzard, all five of us made the fateful journey after nightfall to take the ablutions together in a square unpainted building, and the invigorating, blood-tingling custom probably had much to do with our rugged health and our ability to toil relentlessly from sun to sun. The building was heated by wood all day Saturday till the mass of rock was red hot and the atmosphere inside blazing hot. The eldest girl would go over the body of each bather in the tub with a heavy stiff brush and then with a showering swish of water on the hot rocks change the atmosphere to hot steam which rolled outward from the arch of stones and blotted out everything from sight. The excessive heat, the moisture, opened our pores and the poisons tumbled in little rivulets down our arms and legs. It was wonderful to just stand there and feel the vigor, rather than weakness, build up in the body. Swipes from the long willow switch made our blood tingle with pepped up circulation and then a bucket of chilling water poured over our bodies would close the pores the tremendous heat had opened so widely. It was a distinct shock —but most exhilarating. Each one of us submitted docilely as we knew it was our only protection against colds, chills and chest disturbances. The Saturday Night Bath took a full hour.

Hydrotherapy is the time-tested natural method for restoration of the body's own "radiators" of warmth and invigoration.

This natural healing method helps to increase the speed of circulation, liberate congestion, carry extra blood to the brain, and increase its supply of oxygen and nutrition. By using simple water-packs, fomentations, contrast baths and applications, many common aches and pains can actually be bathed away. Water applications help revive and rejuvenate a sluggish circulation.

I have found that a hot bath, as hot as can be tolerated, relieves headaches, especially migraine. The benefit is to draw the blood away from the whirling, active brain. The heat relaxes the body, untangles the nerves, smoothes out any mix-up in the digestive system and helps us to go to sleep. A hot foot bath will improve the circulation in the feet, the skin and simultaneously revitalize internal organs. It warms the person, helps the person relax and will ease any inflammation in the feet. Soaking an aching and/or swollen foot in hot water for four minutes helps contract the blood vessels and provides a form of increased circulation. After this four minute hot water immersion, remove the foot and soak it in cold water up to one minute. This contrast from hot to cold provides internal exercise to the blood vessels. The hot foot bath should not be given in the presence of blood vessel disease of arms and legs or in the condition of diabetes. Also be careful that the addition of hot water to the tub does not burn the feet.

A fomentation (warm or hot poultice) provides natural and drugless relief to aching, stiffness or pain in the internal organs through the activation of nerve health and in the muscles and joints by stirring up fresh blood supply which soothes inflammation. When there is pain in any part of the body, it indicates that there is some type of congestion in or around the spot. A short hot application, followed by a cold application, provides natural stimulation and is preferred by some specialists because it is relaxing and relieves nervous tension while it brings circulation to the surface of the body. Fomentation also relieves nervous spasms and wrenching pains that make bending over a torturous experience. Use a warm, moist bandage, or the application of a warm wet cloth with a heating pad, but be sure to put a plastic sheet over the wet cloth. This moist heat often ends mysterious aches and pains by helping to stimulate the function of internal organs and also stimulating white blood cell activity.

Fomentation has a sedative effect by drawing the blood away

from the head and internal organs by natural spine-abdomen heat applications. This helps ease aching and stiffness and low back pain. A fomentation on the spine provides healing heat to the little nerve centers in the back, causing a natural flow of blood and feeling of spasm relaxation. The spinal muscles start to relax. A fomentation on the abdomen helps pull out the tension (knots in the stomach) and increase blood circulation. The heat brings extra blood to the skin, drawing it from the inner organs, relieving the internal congestion. Cold compresses to the neck and head constrict the blood vessels to ease the pounding blood flow that causes a feeling of light-headedness. This naural method helps the body stir up its own sluggish healing forces to bring about relief without drugs. Always use warm, moist heat for ailments. If this method does not seem to work, then the cold, most therapy should be utilized. And always remember, no two human beings are alike. What is effective for one person may not work for another. Every plant, animal and human body is different. Therefore, each one must be handled individually.

POSTURE, EXERCISE AND RELAXATION —

Posture is vital to healthful living. Correct posture equalizes and balances the bodily forces, aids circulation and respiration, and brings the spine to its natural curve, thereby increasing vitality, mental alertness and personal efficiency. Good posture establishes a right balance in the psychological functions of the body and aids in the development of greater reserves of nervous energy so that we can absorb the stresses and strains of everyday living more easily.

Let us watch carefully how we stand and sit. A sturdy spruce tree is far more stately than a weeping willow. We should ourselves be the ones to correct this. With good posture, we can enjoy more self-confidence and greater ability to cope with difficult problems. We can better govern and control our own attitudes towards our human and material environment and thereby our reactions to the life around us. We are actors and reactors in and to the life around us. When dealing with other people, good posture makes a far better impression than poor posture. An erect, proud carriage evokes feelings of confidence and vitality in both person and observer.

To begin our day well, we must charge our minds and bodies with such youthful energy that we can go forth into the competitive, hustling world with a natural tranquility and bubbling vigor. Just as we would not start off in our car without giving it a moment to warm up, so we should not plunge carelessly into the day without preparing our mind and body. When we first awaken in the morning, let us lie quietly and ask God to guide us, banish all worries from our minds, feel secure and hold to a positive attitude.

Do not jump directly out of bed. Animals know this instinctively. Watch a cat yawn when rising from her nap, stretch her forepaws as far as they will go, claw the rug with an alternating motion pull herself forward, arch her back and then pull herself back again. There is nothing so good for starting circulation as stretching exercises. Slowly stretching our bodies, catlike, as we lie on our beds, let us yawn and wiggle our toes in one direction and then in the other. And sit up, sit up slowly.

Tight, cramped and kinked muscles in the back of the neck upon awakening can often drain away vital morning energy. To ease these muscles, let's turn our head slowly to the left, then to the right as far as possible; stretch our head slowly to the left, then to the right as far as possible; stretch our heads back as far as possible, breathing in and holding the breath for a moment, and then exhaling slowly as we bend the neck forward as far as possible. If the cords of the neck hurt, rub them vigorously. Then let's relax and drop our chins to our chest. Breathing in, rotate our heads very slowly to the right and straight back: breathing out, rotate our heads to the left and finish with the head hanging limply on our chest, thus making a complete circle with our head, first a clockwise circle, then counterclockwise. The neck roll will loosen up stiff neck muscles. We should feel a pleasant pull as we stretch those tensed up neck and shoulder muscles. Let's perform each of these exercises seven times.

To healthfully speed up circulation and lubricate wrists and limbs, somewhat stiff from lying still through the night, let's try this "warming up" exercise. Shaking our hands and wrists loosely before us, as fast and vigorously as possible, continuing until we have a flexible or well-lubricated up-and-down movement. Let's imagine our hands are wet and we are trying to shake away the drops of moisture. When we get out of bed, we can put a spring into our step by vigorously awakening our legs; shaking our left leg with a loose, flexible leg and ankle motion. Let's kick and shake our hip and knee joint to bring the oxygen-carrying blood to the tips of our toes. Now let's repeat with our right leg.

For an electrifying awakening, we can place our hands in a sink filled with cold water. Keeping the spine straight, we inhale deeply through the nostrils and exhale through the mouth, emptying the lungs. Repeat seven times. Deep breathing will awaken us and banish drowsiness.

These natural laws for rising in the morning help oxygenate our systems, flush our wastes and invigorate the mind and body. To benefit, we should do these exercises every morning, for as we fit them into our schedules, they will require just ten golden minutes in the morning to add up ten golden hours of better energy. This is a good time to practice zone therapy on our feet with golf balls or a coke bottle. We are now ready for our two glasses of warm water. These may be taken pure or with the juice of one lemon, making sure the water has been neutralized with wheatgrass.

Life and exercise go hand in hand. The normal body cannot achieve its goals without proper exercise. Languor and the lack of desire to exercise do not mean laziness so much as sickness and improper nutrition which slows down the circulation. The lazy person is a sick person, exactly as the alcoholic or drug user is a sick person.

There are many types of exercises, from the strenuous calisthenics to the placid exercises of the Yogis. Yogic exercises are of a different character and have a different end in view from the more strenuous setting-up exercises. The ends sought in Hatha Yoga are an augmented flow of oxygen into the system and the elimination of carbon dioxide gas, the cleansing and vitalizing of the digestive tract, and the gaining of complete muscular control, including the involuntary muscles. Directly or indirectly, they are cleansing in their nature and the practice of these exercises is conducive to health and longevity. It regulates the action of the heart, lungs and brain. It promotes digestion and circulation of the blood. It helps to remove impurities in the blood stream, and so enable one to possess a high standard of health, vigor and vitality.

The following exercises should be practiced daily to the extent determined by our time, our strength and our disposition toward them. We should approach our exercises with more than willingness, with zest, for they will do us good largely according to the amount of pleasure we derive from them. We should set aside a special time each day and give ourselves wholly to them. And let's not watch the clock; boredom and impatience are obstacles to progress. The best time to practice is in the early morning. For those who find the exercises flow more easily in the evening, be sure to wait at least three hours after eating a normal meal. Practice in a quiet room where there is plenty of fresh air, lightly clad so that clothes do not restrict movement, breathing or blood flow. A pad or cushion, or a folded blanket, about the size of a single bed, is preferred by many people. The exercises should be done calmly, with patience and determination and strictly without any attitude of competition.

In the beginning, each exercise should be repeated two—three times. In general we exhale when bending forward and inhale when bending backward, and breathe calmly, rhythmically while maintaining the pose. Forceful breathing or holding the breath in the pose may be harmful. We should rest after each pose as long as we need, and breathing the heartbeat should return to normal before doing the next exercise. Vigorous types of exercise should be followed by ten minutes of corpse pose or deep relaxation.

The reduction of the belly and the strengthening of the muscles of the waist and abdomen are so important that there are many exercises involving the raising of the arms above the head. There is nothing so good for circulation as stretching exercises. For this first exercise, we stand comfortably, and relaxed, arms at sides. Gently and cheerfully, let's lift our arms toward the sky, palms facing forward. Then, gracefully and slowly, bending forward at the waist, let's slowly, very slowly, bring our hands down in an arc in front of us to reach for our toes, keeping our knees straight and following with our head.

Do not strain. Eventually our palms can be placed flat on the floor in front of our feet and the forehead will touch the knees or legs. Until we are that limber, as we will become if we practice these exercises regularly, either remain leaning forward with the arms stretching toward the floor, or grasp the calves or ankles and *gently* draw the head closer to the legs, being careful not to strain. Be sure to move in and out of this slowly, gracefully. Beginners hold five to ten minutes.

WAIST ROLL: Standing with feet comfortably apart for balance, hands on hips or waist, let's bend forward slightly at the waist, inclining head. Slowly, very slowly, rotate to the right, always bending or moving from the waist, and slowly, very slowly, complete a circle with the upper portion of the body, keeping head in line with inclination of body. Do three times in clockwise direction, enlarging the circle with each rotation; then three times in reverse direction.

Now sit down in a comfortable position and relax a few moments. This is a good time to do some eye exercises or the neck roll for relaxation.

POSTERIOR STRETCH: Sitting with our legs together in front of us, let's stretch our arms above and behind us, leaning back to follow their path as far as we can without losing balance. Or we may begin by lying on our backs on the floor with arms stretched over our heads and then raise ourselves slightly from the floor, holding position a few inches off the floor. Until our stomach muscles become stronger and can hold and balance us, we can have our arms stretched in front of us for balance position and then stretch them back over our heads before rising up further, if necessary lying back down. Now let's slowly raise our body to a sitting position, bringing our arms forward in an arc, toward our toes, continuing to bend forward until we rest our hands on our ankles or feet, or as far down on our legs as we can comfortably reach while keeping legs straight. Gently, slowly, bending the elbows, we incline our head and shoulders toward our knees, still keeping legs straight, and hold for count of ten. Then gently, steadily, with an even motion, let's straighten our arms and reach further for our toes, being careful not to strain or overreach ourselves. There should not be any jerky bounces, but peaceful, steady effort.

Eventually, when we are very much more limber, our forehead will touch the knees. Hold extended pose for count of 10 and then slowly and smoothly straighten up and sit back. Repeat two times. This exercise reduces fat, stimulates digestion fire and is useful in enlargement of the spleen.

COBRA: We begin by lying flat on the floor on our stomachs, arms resting comfortably by our sides, legs together and head resting on chin or turned to the side and resting on cheek. With head facing in a straight line with the body, slowly, very slowly, let's begin raising head and shoulders, leading with the back of the head, as far as possible without assistance. Then placing palms on the floor, approximately below shoulders, fingers spread and facing together or front, continue to slowly, very slowly raise upper portion of the body from the waist as far as possible without assistance, like a serpent, to get head and shoulders as high as possible without putting weight on hands.

Then using arms for assistance, slowly straighten elbows. Let's continue to raise upper portion of the body as far as is comfortable, pushing from the hands and letting the body from the navel downward to the toes remain touching the ground. We must be careful not to strain or push too far, such that there is any pain in the back. This should be done with an even, graceful steady motion, breathing gently and deeply. Hold top position for 10 seconds and then slowly, very slowly, we will lower ourselves back down, first using hands for assistance, then without hands. The entire exercise should be a fluid graceful motion. Repeat two or three times. This exercise is excellent for the digestive system and for expelling gas.

BICYCLE: Turn over and after resting, we will begin this exercise lying on our backs with hands resting comfortably at our sides. We slowly raise our legs until they make a right angle with the ground, then pressing against the floor with the palms of the hands, we will slowly, very slowly, continue to raise legs and hips until they are pointing vertically upward or slanting diagonally over our heads for ease in lifting and balance. The body is raised sufficiently high to allow the chest to press against the chin and supported with the two hands at the back or on the hips. Now, with the help of the forearms as a support and elbows planted firmly on the ground, let's pretend we are riding a bicycle and energetically paddle with legs in the air.

The Western idea of physical culture is the kind of bodily activity involving a kind of competence, endurance and muscular efficiency, in such things like walking, running, swimming, skating and the like. Let's drop the competence and enjoy these recreational activities as they were intended—for health and recreation. Benjamin Franklin maintained that swimming was one of the most healthful and agreeable exercises in the world. Dick Gregory, who has been on a juice fast for more than a year, runs miles each day, laughing and growing stronger.

This is a good point to begin a detailed examination of how to live better for less, for the automobile is way ahead of every other flagrant money waster in our lives. Let's learn to walk and re-experience our youth and relearn patterns of living that don't involve the automobile. Neighborhoods haven't vanished since our childhood; our orientations have just overstepped their boundaries. On our daily walks, we will return to a pattern where relationships are once more on a human basis. There are actually people along the way. Animals, too. I used to have a regular morning session with a couple of squirrels in the park who would meet me chattering madly on their hind feet. And in the evening, going home from work, I would have a pleasant chat in the Shortcut with a beautiful gray tabby who lived there.

We can get further into the spirit of things by doing most of our shopping on foot and using the bus lines for short trips that are outside the immediate neighborhood. Many of the things we habitually go downtown or to a favorite store across town for we will find right in our own neighborhood, when we begin to develop a sense of identity with the shops in our area. Suddenly we are no longer living in a metropolis, but in a community. Our basic horizons will pull back and we will begin to feel a closeness to the neighborhood we call home. Walking will put us in good condition to start bicycle riding for business as well as pleasure. With a bicycle, our neighborhood will expand from one mile to several and we'll find ourselves seldom taking the bus anymore, except when weather dictates. A bike carrier with a few straps will hold a surprising lot, whether big packages from a shopping spree with the money saved on gas, parking, etc., or a picnic basket for a day in the country.

There are many delightful things that can be done with a touring bicycle; long weekend rides in the country, camping vacations, hosteling in certain areas, air-freighting bicycle and self to faraway places, etc. Canada and most of Europe have free hostels across the country—in every major city and town. Dr. Paul Dudley White of Boston, world's leading heart specialist, considers bicycling one of the best forms of exercise. Bicycles are a popular form of transportation as well as pleasurable exercises for all ages in many European countries. Most of Scandinavia boasts a ratio of one bicycle for every two inhabitants. This country, too, was going in that direction before we became crazy about power and "progress".

In China, they do not even have private cars on the streets —only buses and bicycles. Why wait for such a restriction? We all realize that something must be done to alleviate the pollution and congestion in our cities. Why not start now, voluntarily, to bring about this change through a bicycling program and at the same time discover new health, a more human perspective and personal kind of freedom. It is not too late to rebuild strong and healthy bodies capable of undertaking such a program. I have had a great deal of experience with folks who lack energy, folks even so weak that they cannot walk around the house and are bedridden. After being nourished entirely on living food for only three weeks, these same people found themselves capable to walking two or three miles without tiring. Organically grown, living uncooked food can give us plenty of energy for healthful, pleasant modes of transportation and recreation.

RELAXATION —

People who have mastered the simple art of relaxed living in this tense world have prepared themselves temperamentally to grow quickly and pleasantly into emotional maturity, to become the balanced individuals for which we all have the natural equipment. Cares, difficulties, problems, pressures are inherent to modern living and are the breeders of tension, which medical authorities agree is the cause of a great many illnesses and diseases, sickness with a myriad of symptoms. Tension is our worst enemy as it wastes precious energy and health and destroys happiness and the joy of living.

When we are at our wit's end and everything seems to have turned against us, instead of doggedly carrying on the fight with depleted strength, we should seize the opportunity to relax. Later we will return to action revitalized and invigorated. If we really lay aside our disturbances and cares for just 30 minutes and sink ourselves into deep relaxation with entire concentration, we will be better able to deal with them when we have been renewed and refreshed with deep relaxation. But it must be *deep* relaxation, not just ordinary relaxation, if we would experience the full, refreshing boost.

Deep relaxation means relieving the mind and body of all conscious tension and contraction. The original interpretation, "to loosen or slacken", makes much more sense than the modern idea of "relaxing" by substituting one type of hustle for another. Deep relaxation enables us to "let go" as many muscles as possible and as many thoughts as possible, to let the body and brain slump completely—an attitude, if you like, of complete resignation.

Even the ordinary dog and cat have survived domesticity to the extent of retaining their powers of deep relaxation. Our pets are indeed expert at relaxing. A dog moves round in circles preparatory to flopping on the floor, his body becomes a dead weight, every muscle is placed completely at ease. And, like all animals, he very sensibly favors the horizontal position —lying down. Although even in the deepest stages of relaxation there is always a residue of muscular contraction, naturally this is more pronounced when the muscles have to hold the body up.

The ideal hour to do deep relaxation is just after coming home from work and before the heavy meal of the day, be that evening, noon or morning. Just before bed is not a good time, for deep relaxation will give so much energy and vitality that it may become impossible then to go to sleep. The only equipment needed is a quiet room where we will not be interrupted for any reason short of an emergency and 30 minutes of time. We must banish any idea of hurry, and any idea of effort, and take our time doing this routine. The whole purpose of this experiment is to acquaint all the muscles of our body with the difference of the feeling of tension and the feeling of relaxation, to teach our bodies and minds what relaxation is, thereby making it possible for relaxation to enter. We alternately tense and relax each and every part of our body, individually, starting from the toes, alternately relaxing and tensing the muscles in every part working up from the feet to the top of the head. We must be as neutral in mind as we can make ourselves be, letting our whole being faithfully register every sensation and welcome any pleasurable experience that might result.

When we have worked on every part of our body, let's rest and breathe deeply, gently, rhythmically, enjoying the completely relaxed feeling of all the muscles of our bodies. Staying quiet and continuing deep, rhythmic breathing until our spouse or roommate, or the alarm tells us it's time to return to the normal affairs of the day. Then we will rouse ourselves slowly, catlike, from a pleasant drowsiness, while reveling in deep relaxation. As we pick up our kitbag of cares, difficulties, problems and troubles that we left outside the door, we will find it feels not quite as heavy as when we left it there. Because of a greater confidence, from being relaxed mentally and physically, we will be better able to cope with the problems that life will continue to lay at our door. If we practice deep relaxation before mealtime, we will find that we will eat more slowly, more leisurely and our food tastes better and digests better because of our slower and relaxed eating. We should take time to enjoy our food.

As we continue this program for 30 days, we will become more and more relaxed, less irritable, less prone to flares of anger, more like what people call "an easy person to get along with". General health will improve, we will have more energy for work and play and will experience a real zest for living. We will be able to accomplish more and do better work with less effort and without strain or tension. Ideas will come more readily how to solve problems, etc. We will feel many years younger than before our first experience with deep relaxation.

SLEEP —

One of the most important and basic laws of abundantly healthful living is a good night's sleep. Sleep is a natural function of all living things. The length of sleep required to insure adequate rest for the body varies and each person's requirements are different. An elderly person who does not do heavy work and rests a lot does not require much sleep. Children who eat live, healthful foods and have good elimination are filled with energy and will not sleep very long. When children are stuffed with unnatural, cooked foods, constipation results, causing the overtaxed, toxious body to require longer hours of unnatural sleep. Persons who are calm and cheerful and work very hard actually use very little physical energy and need little sleep. It is the toxins created in the body by violent or oppressive emotions and by bad food that tires the body and creates the need for long hours of rest. At the same time, it is impossible for them to fall asleep which forces them to take sleeping pills, etc. By doing our work with a cheerful disposition, with a sense of pride and accomplishment, even though it may be very strenuous or even tedious, we feel uplifted and sleep well and feel rested. People who worry about getting too little sleep and who are taking sleeping pills obtain very little of the right kind of sleep. The mind may become unconscious, but their body is not resting; it is busy working to fight off toxic effects of these unnatural substances. Though these persons may "sleep" for many hours, they obtain little actual rest.

When we sleep, our bedroom should not be heated and we should sleep with the windows open whenever possible. Adopt the good habit of breathing through the nose; this helps us avoid dryness of the throat and snoring. Good ventilation is of utmost importance. Our bed should not be placed in a recess or surrounded by curtains which impede the flow of air. A firm bed is best and the coverings should be light and warm. Avoid heavy and close night attire; it is best to sleep without it. Our skin needs to breathe while we sleep. We should not leave the light on in our room at night as it will tire our eyes, and we should not go to bed until at least two hours after dinner.

The most healthful sleeping position is on the right side. This position promotes natural sleep with little effort and does not impede the beating of the heart. And while we are in this position, the work of the heart, lungs and stomach is relaxed as they are on top of the other organs. The American Indians used this traditional health law for generations and they still follow it in our modern times, enjoying refreshing sleep.

Relaxation is the essence of a good night's sleep. It calls for natural and drugless methods of providing the mind and body with a healthful desire to go to sleep refreshed. A charged-up brain and nervous system has to be relaxed before it can let us sleep. Therefore, we should prepare ourselves for refreshing sleep with gentle persuasion. Forget all about the hustle and bustle of the day and sink into a state of complete passivity and sleep will enfold us. When we lie down, divert our thoughts from business and family worries, our minds from disharmonious things, for these provoke a disturbed night's sleep.

Deep breathing is very relaxing. This rhythmic breathing provides internal ventilation and eliminates harsh irritants that may grate the nerves and deprive us of restful sleep. Deep breathing exercises help to melt tensions and offer relaxation and rejuvenating sleep. The benefits of soothing water to provide healthful sleep is well known. The natural tonic of a comfortably warm bath is one of the oldest and best remedies for loosening tight, tense muscles. A brief nap a few hours before bedtime, or deep relaxation after a day's work and before dinner, can help relax our brains and nervous system and create a state of euphoria that is a natural sleep-inducer when we finally get into bed at our scheduled bedtime.

Researchers have found that much sleeplessness can be traced to staring even when the eyelids are shut! Hydrotherapy, is a natural law of relaxation, including eye relaxation. Apply comfortably hot water to the closed eyes and follow with an application of comfortably cold water. This helps flush out impurities and dilate clogged arteries, promoting circulation to sluggish channels that force the eye to start wide open even though the lids are closed in sought-for sleep.

There is a wise saying about sleep: "He who would be healthy in the morning must prepare like a camel at bedtime to have his burdens lifted. For to the unburdened, the night will be bright as stardust. For sleep is a gentle maid, beautiful as an angel, who brings her lovely wares for the one who rests without anxiety, safe and secure."

MASSAGE, ZONE THERAPY AND ACUPUNCTURE

Healing with the hands is as old as the human being's aches and pains and was known to the ancient Chinese, Egyptians and Grecians. The "laying on of the hands" is mentioned in the Scriptures and its beneficial effects have been recognized in many passages. My work with the sick has convinced me that the laying on of hands can send powerful energizing rays into a disturbed body. Over and over again, I have seen a transmission of healing power from a normal body into a sick one. In several instances, I am certain that dying persons have been so strengthened by these healing rays that they attained a new lease on life.

The blood is the circulating life force. The nerves, capillaries, lymph, arteries, skin, etc., are the channels through which this life force harmoniously flows. However, lymph and blood and nerve impulses can flow freely only through unobstructed channels. All the organs have nerve and capillary outlets to the skin surface to participate in the cosmic forces of the universe. If they're blocked, this life force is blocked and we become sick. We are not in harmony with Mother Nature. We need to clean our blood stream with living, uncooked, organically grown nutriments.

Massage, spot therapy, acupuncture, reflexology, contact healing, chiropracty, and osteopathy are the great means for releasing this congestion of these parts, increasing the circulation and raising body vitality. And as the vitality increases, Nature has the strength to overcome and throw off the poisons of the system. Through manipulation and/or applied pressure, pain can be relieved and help to restore health to any part of the body. The most attractive element of such therapy is that we can heal ourselves and others through the use of our hands.

Massage is the rubbing, stroking, kneading or tapping of the flesh with the bare hands, the working of the hands onto the skin with a firm pressure, in a rhythmical pattern. The Greeks, Germans and Swedes were among the first to use this direct, on-the-body contact on their people. This rhythmical pattern can produce an acceleration in the blood to improve circulation, relax the nerves and loosen any tension in the muscle structure, which if not worked out will in time impair the body's health. The strokes and movements on the skin help to break up the fatty tissues that are of no use to the body, to strengthen the muscles and tone up the areas of the body which have been neglected by the lack of exercise. Massage has positive effects on the nervous system, relieving muscle spasms. It also increases the elimination process by helping the lungs, kidneys and colon to eliminate toxins so that the body will function at its normal capacity. When we are feeling tired and numb, self-massage can help bring the body awake.

A severe headache may have nothing to do with any damage afflicting the head; instead the source of the trouble may be the stomach or the colon. In 1913 William H. Fitzgerald, M.D., discovered that "there are ten invisible currents through the body". He described ten longitudinal zones, five on each side of the body, extending from the head, through the trunk, to the toes and fingers. When an organ malfunctions, points along its meridian will become painful and hard, even before the organ itself aches. The meridian network just below the skin is actually an integral part of the body's control mechanism and defense medium, regulating the body. Neatly aligned along our body's meridians are the numerous pressure point eyes. Dr. Fitzgerald found on the surface of the body these pin point areas, tender or painful to touch. Pressure on these areas can break up crystalline waste deposits, increasing nerve and blood supply to relieve congestion in corresponding areas in the same zone, however distant the affliction from the area where pressure is applied. It can speed the detoxification process and strengthen internal organs.

Eunice Inham Stepfel perfected compression massage of the feet. She feels that since there are reflex points in the feet corresponding to every part of the body it is sufficient to work on the feet alone.

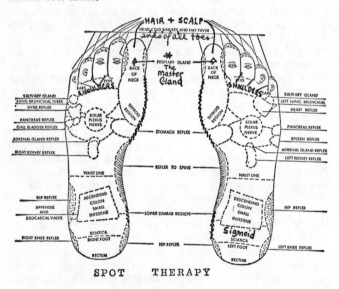

SPOT THERAPY

Nothing can bring on old age more quickly than the abuse of the feet through over-weight, high heels, cramped toes and improper diet. Meet all uncomfortable foot conditions by soaking them in hot water once or twice a day for 15 minutes, by changing the diet to living food and by utilizing zone therapy. Press the foot with your thumb on any part designated here as infuencing some other place in the body. Two persons can accomplish wonders by working on each other's feet at the same time.

Just as pressure on certain spots in the feet can have beneficial results in various parts of the body, so also may pressure on certain bones of the spine likewise have healthful reactions on the various muscles and organs. This pressure routine on the spine and the routine for regaining normal health is now officially recognized and widely used throughout the world.

Spot therapy is useful to relieve tension, pains, aches and discomfort associated with dietary transition. It works far better than any known chemical painkiller and produces no complications. The results are often visible after a single 20-minute application, although at the start only temporary relief can be anticipated. Pain will persist until the cause—congestion caused by the present, constipating nourishment—has been eliminated. Seldom is only one organ affected; generally it is a total body emergency and some conditions require many months of work before one can obtain the desired results.

Migraine headaches are a sign of indigestion. They usually originate in the colon or stomach. Sweet food combined with starches can cause fermentation, producing in the stomach a wide range of toxins. The task of eliminating them so overtaxes the liver and kidneys that the endocrine glands overwork in an attempt to direct the toxins to other eliminative organs. This hyperfunction can cause the pituitary glands to swell and press against their enclosure, sometimes causing the severe pain of migraine headaches (*Food Is Your Best Medicine,* H. Bieler, M.D.). Zone therapy at the earliest sign of indigestion, anger, tightness in the neck, pain in the eyeballs, soreness in the re- flex areas related to the digestive system, can prevent head- aches. If the headache is the result of protein indulgence, sometimes ¼ glass of very warm lemon water or fresh pine- apple juice is helpful.

Spot therapy works on all reflex points on the face and feet, with 90% of time on points corresponding to the ascending, transverse and descending colon, the small intestines and the stomach, can relieve constipation. After a twenty-minute application, there will be a bowel movement within an hour, although severe cases might require two applications of spot therapy.

Sleeplessness and tension are a sign of indigestion, constipation, severe cleansing reactions or emotional stress; work on the reflex points as for headache and constipation can relieve symptoms and after five minutes of intensive work, the person will probably fall asleep.

Acupuncture is the ancient Chinese method of treating pain and disease by puncturing the body with needles, inserting usually silver and gold needles into the points of the meridian corresponding to the malfunctioning organs or parts of the body. In 1929, the Chinese condemned their ancient medicine and decided to go all out Western, but in the past decade or so the pendulum has swung the other way and acupuncture is now being emphasized. Most of China's Western-trained physicians have gone back to school to learn the ancient technique of acupuncture, while *The Chinese Medical Journal* recently reported that acupuncture is good for some 200 diseases, including appendicitis and infantile paralysis.

MUSIC, ASTROLOGY, MEDITATION and SOLUITUDE

Music has a tremendous influence on the spirit. Because it is creative, it can raise the human mind to the portals of heaven or bring it to the very depths of hell. Good music can liberate the emotions of the spirit and bring us in tune with all things in life that are harmonious. It helps us to flow smoothly with the current of life rather than against it. When I say "good music", I mean uplifting music which is soothing and gives peace and I have found that music that is light and simple is best for uplifting the human mind.

I once heard a teacher from India tell of a sanitarium in a small village in his homeland where all therapy was administered in the form of music. The results, as he related them, were miraculous in cases where the physical disturbances in the body were based on nerve depletion, excess emotionalism and other factors in the nervous system. The physicians of the ancient great civilizations maintained that the body was a symphony of vibrations and that music could help to break up disease and bring the body back into harmony. They used music for many different illnesses. Scientists have discovered that even plants respond to music. In this country we are rapidly adopting the therapeutic properties of music. Employers are discovering that music improves the disposition of their employees, resulting in better work performance. The greatest aid we can give to a sick person on the road to recovery is to take his or her mind away from the pain. I ask these people to listen to music or to get into a tub of warm water and relax.

Our modern music has contributed much to the problems of a sick society, as it degrades the mentality and helps to ruin the physical body. It is difficult for parents to remove this type of music from children, but by having plenty of good music around and, most important, by giving love and understanding, parents can quietly replace even the desire for the discordant, degenerating music. These young people are our future citizens and I know how sincere they are. Their greatest desire is to be of service to humanity. Children who show a particular interest in music should be encouraged to develop that talent. In talking with a great many hippies, I have learned that in most cases their parents had misunderstood their motives and their natural talents were suppressed. Their inharmonious music is their expression of their anguish and despair. Many have gone so far overboard in their angry, rebellious methods of living that bad nutrition and harmful drugs have ruined their health. We can help them regain their emotional and physical well being. These young people need encouragement and understanding through which they may be brought back to a harmonious life.

ASTROLOGY —

Because of the tremendous help and guidance it offers us, I have been interested in astrology for many years. Astrology is an instrument of knowledge, the algebra of life. Like mathematics, astrology has no meaning in and of itself. The symbols of the different planets and signs, just like the numbers in math, have no significance unless related to the whole, to the individual and group context of our lives. Working practically with these symbols can give us invaluable information about our physical, emotional, mental and spiritual make-up.

Contrary to popular opinion, astrology is not fortune-telling, for it points out choices we have to make, not static conditions over which we have no control. It's greatest help lies in showing us crossroads we will come to and patterns and conditions that exist with which we have to work and to choose from. And it emphasizes the timely importance of these choices by showing us that these crossroads do not happen every day and the choices, therefore, are not always available to us. Astrology deals with the individual vibrations of which each of us is made. It shows us our personality limitations and strengths and areas in our make-up of which we might not be aware otherwise, areas which could point out new directions, subconscious problems coming out in veiled ways, unknown strengths and weaknesses. But most important, astrology shows us how we fit into the whole.

I have always had a great desire to help humanity, but my many weaknesses, both known to me and hidden within from me, prevented me from going forward and serving as I deserved. The understanding I gained through astrology, which not only defines these weak points but teaches us how to deal with them and reveals to us the hidden strengths in our characters with which we can combat them, enabled me to work harder and overcome these difficulties. The average Pisces tends to be a dreamer, to see life from a spiritual viewpoint to the neglect of the physical, which usually manifests as a very weak digestion and did in myself, also preventing me from much work. Pisces tends to be a dual personality, one day very sad and the next day joyful, letting the emotions overpower common sense and often thinking people are taking advantage of us. Pisces is very sensitive to the feelings of other persons and seeks to escape from any conflict, and to drown problems in pleasure or alcohol or drugs, rather than making the effort to meet with and improve the situation. Pisces is a great procrastinator, a "do it tomorrow" person, always bemoaning the fact that "everything happens to me", and of never having an opportunity to improve matters.

Through great suffering and discipline and poverty, I was forced to turn to God fully for direction and help. This gave me strength to write because it made me understand that everything has to come from within, and that there is no reason for seeking to conceal the truth. Now I can truly say my character has changed diametrically from what it was before, although of course there is still much to be done until I can fully fill the place the Almighty intended me to occupy.

This "language of the stars" takes a while to sink into the subconscious, which is where it has to be in order to strengthen our intuition. To gain as much benefit as possible takes many hours of study and meditation, and a lot of time for the newly learned language and knowledge to sink in. It is wise to remember that anything negative we might instill or stir up in other people when reading their charts we are responsible for karmically; the power of suggestion is not to be fooled around with. We cannot be too careful when dealing with people's lives! There are too many people who read one book and set themselves up as astrologers, with little knowledge of the subject. Astrology is something to be taken seriously, just as psychology and psycho-therapy. Many young astrologers will fall by the wayside when they are put into situations where they must follow all their own advice, be proof of their teachings by their own life example.

Astrology is a new age science and a very valuable tool for those who know how to use it. It is coming more and more into its own, and every day more people are using this science to set up weddings, time of conception, opening of shops and businesses, and, most important, for self-knowledge. Remember, astrology is merely a way of tuning in, of coming out of our separate spokes into the great wheel of Life and uniting with our brothers and sisters with the awe and love which is our birthright. All our differences are merely different roads traveling to and from the center. Astrology is a way of seeing that we are all the same, of learning about individual selves and taking care of business so that we can receive God's Love and Light and Help. It is a way of finding all of Life within us.

Astrology is also a very effective tool in healing, as the energies of all the planets are tied up with the glands and circulation. It can help us discover the *root* cause of our own or another's true illness, as well as bodily weaknesses. The stars suggest or indicate a way out of any predicament or problem, but the choice always remains our own.

"O Solitude! Where are thy own charms." This was the spontaneous flow of expression from a poet when he was one with nature—sentiments of the sublime and the beautiful. Once we have tasted properly, to the very depths of our being, the happiness of solitude, we will never leave it at any cost. Its soothing and soul-elevating vibrations must be felt for us to understand the beauty and peace of solitude. The spiritual vibratory condition, this glandeur and benign influence, are within each one of us, if we will only search for this remarkable place.

The word "soul" is derived from Sol (sun) and, just as the sun is the light center of this universe, the soul is the light-center of our being. Psychology has learned that our mental activity is not limited to one plane of consciousness and indeed our conscious life is in reality but a reflection of our deeper interior mental and spiritual activity. The living cells and tiny organisms which compose our physical bodies are influenced especially by radiations from our own minds, from our "souls", as well as from the atmosphere and invisible planes around us.

Under the disturbing influences and conditions of the Aquarian Age, we are being constantly bombarded by new ideas, unique suggestions, unforeseen problems and difficulties. Some are trivial, some overpowering. We can complain bitterly and blame others for our discomfort, or we can learn to meditate, to relax our bodies and calm our minds and find peace within. The more stress we have in life, the greater is the need for solitude, for seeking guidance from within. In solitude we can acquire real peace of mind. Let me share several meditations I've learned.

We need a quiet, comfortable, cheerful space to sit or lie down. Relaxation in body and mind is prerequisite. We must be thankful and avoid negative thinking that lowers our vibrations. As we lie quietly, let us hum the "OMMMM" long and drawn out, repeating three times. Nothing can restrain us but ourselves, so proceed without fear. We need patience and a keen desire for health and joy—God's gifts if only we will claim them. Thus we utilize the unlimited help we can receive only from God within.

Gather daily for meditation. I have proved over and over again that nothing is impossible if we are willing to be guided.

However, we must make an effort and muster patience and have faith that help will come. If it does not come, we alone are blocking the way. We must let go of all selfishness and adopt a loving attitude. There is a solution to every problem, but every wish must be backed by honest effort and strong will. If we abide by Nature's laws, health, happiness, and peace will be ours. But to follow these laws, we must have a desire to do so, be willing to work, and above all possess faith.

We can prove for ourselves the value of praise by praising someone we have long criticized. Notice the change, not only in ourselves but in the person praised. Why do so many children resent their parents? Rather than giving praise for their successes and understanding for their failures, parents demand success, offering empty material bribes, and give caustic criticism and discouragement for failure. Praise, like interchange with our Heavenly Father, would produce in children love and gratitude toward their parents.

Above all, learn patience. We must learn to love not only ourselves but friends and even enemies. Whenever we recall someone who has treated us wrongly, bless that person. We must forgive ourselves as well as all others. To develop an understanding heart, let's imagine ourselves in the other's place—practice the Golden Rule. When we cringe at another's foolishness, recall now flowers grow and bloom, silently. All Nature unfolds gradually and gratefully like the lotus. Be thou patient.

Remember, we are needed by the Almighty. The Almighty works through us, and each one of us can become His instrument. We can become powerhouses for healing and problem solving; we can purify our minds and bodies, the holy temples in which He dwells. Through daily meditation we can condition ourselves to serve Him. At the Mansion, we meditate each day; this helps us to move faster to help sick humanity.

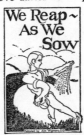

Part IV

Tips For
Every Day Living

HOW TO BEAT THE HIGH COST OF LIVING

We all complain about the high cost of living. Folks generally believe their only escape from this difficulty is to increase their earnings. Few people recognize that as income increases costs rise proportionately. The only practical way to end inflation is to reduce the cost of living. Numerous families have come to the Mansion to learn how they might live on less than a dollar a day. This is not wishful thinking. Anyone can learn these principles in their own home.

Food is our most expensive living requirement, both costly and generally inadequate for proper nutrition. Most diets consist of dead nutrition, which causes premature old age and bodily ailments, mental and spiritual upsets, etc. Fundamentally, our entire system of nourishment needs overhaul. Live food reduces the cost by about three-fourths.

The produce one would need to healthfully feed one person for one week and its cost are as follows: 2 lbs. of wheat (40c), 1 lb. sesame seeds ($1.40), 7 tsp. of kelp (16c), 2 lbs buckwheat seed (40c), and 1 lb of mung beans ($1.40). Adding a variety of fruit ($5.00), the total cost is $8.76 per week, or $1.26 per day.

After one pound of seeds has grown, in a period of five to eight days, the total represents 6 lbs. of solid, live food. One pound of dry wheat can be converted into 2 lbs. of sprouts for cereal or "milk", 4 pounds of wheatgrass, or 42 ounces of enzyme-rich rejuvelac, and is an excellent source of Vitamin B Complex and Vitamin E. Two pounds of buckwheat seed can be converted into 6 lbs. of buckwheat lettuce and 1 lb. of mung beans into 6 lbs. of sprouts for a "complete meal" salad.

Chapter 6 in Part II tells how to grow wheatgrass and buckwheat lettuce, and Chapters 3 and 4 of Part II explain how to sprout and to prepare wonderful dishes from these foods. Food should be eaten uncooked since heat destroys or negates more than 80 per cent of its value.

Yearly style obsolescence probably accounts for 60 per cent of this enormous cost. The vast majority of otherwise intelligent women accept like sheep the stylist's lead. We forget that we know intuitively what remnant is most suitable. A woman's wardrobe should be carefully chosen for appropriate colors, wrinkle-proof and durable materials. The simpler the wardrobe, the easier life becomes. Shoes should be comfortable and low heels worn as much as possible. Each community should run a clothing exchange where women could sell unneeded garments and purchase those they need. Such an establishment could gradually acquire a large selection of quality clothing at reasonable prices.

Do we need two cars in the garage? Sell one and buy a bicycle. And walk more; it's good for our health. Don't buy new cars; recycle. Buy a good used car and save on taxes and insurance. If we live in the city, we can forget that unnecessary car. I found it a real blessing when my car was stolen. Subways and taxis are convenient and reasonable, but walking is always more beautiful.

Our present health insurance is very costly and still it does not cover every contingency. For example, our late President Eisenhower, a veteran, was naturally taken to a veterans' hospital to curtail expenses. Still, his additional expenses at the hospital amounted to about $90,000. Many hospitals now charge the average patient as much as $100 per day. Additionally, we must not overlook the time wasted in hospitals in both suffering and intense worry for the whole family.

Our best health insurance is to work closely with Mother Nature and to adopt Her living, uncooked food diet. Thus we eliminate sickness and disease. We can begin at once to draw upon the wisdom within and become our own doctor, minister and psychiatrist. I recall one woman who stayed at the Mansion. She had pinpointed 31 distinct afflictions. Yet all these upsets magically disappeared when she religiously followed the methods of Mother Nature instead of drugs and artificial remedies.

Beauty costs are tremendously expensive. Why purchase what we can create? Permanent waves are costly and often ruin the hair. After six years of attending to my own hair, I visited the beauty shop for a hair treatment and my hair began to turn gray. I prepare facial creams at home and find them superior to any I can buy. I will gladly send the recipies for these. I have prepared a sheet on how to eliminate wrinkles, how to maintain hair and how to reduce. Send a self-addressed, stamped envelope and donation and I will gladly mail you copies.

Investigate the low-cost educational loans available to our children. Our teens should definitely work during the summer vacation to contribute toward their education. They will learn to appreciate what they have. Cause and effect rule our lives. Our deeds, both good and bad, return our way. All should learn this law when young.

Solar rays offer a vital energy source, which has been neglected and suppressed. Why waste solar energy on destructive purposes, such as the atomic bomb? Let's research construction uses. Let's write to our Congressmen asking why solar energy is not utilized for heating homes, propelling transportation, etc.

Here are some very simple economizing hints for the home:

1. Dry clean our own clothes. Coin machine cleaning will cost one-fifth the dry cleaner's prices.

2. Save on electricity. Turn off lights, television, and other electric appliances when not in use.

3. Save on newspapers, periodicals, and so forth, visit the library.

4. Cut our husbands and children's hair. With practice, we can do as well as any barber.

5. Learn to say "no" to our children if they demand toys and other unnecessary extras. Discipline and appreciation are the greatest gifts we can bestow upon our children.

Under no circumstances seek something for nothing. In the long run, this may prove most expensive.

WOMEN'S CORNER —

Former Secreaty of Health, Education and Welfare, John W. Gardner, steadfastly believes, "The reason why the United States is coming apart at the seams is because most of us pursue selfish interests." Many fervently wish a better world, but few take *personal* responsibility. Patriotism and cooperation have fallen into disrepute. We blame others for our shortcomings; like ostriches, we bury our heads in the sand to suppress the painful truth. Our lives cry for house cleaning; our society for new leadership to provide social, physical and health reform. Whence our salvation?

Men govern all sectors, yet women dominate the Census. Wars, economic disequilibrium, our discontent youth share common roots in imbalance. Might not a more proportionate representation of women and men in seats of power govern our country in peace, understanding and prosperity? As light requires both positive and negative polarity, women, life-bearing motherhood, gentle governess of the home, offsets Man, the traditional warmaker. Mothers naturally oppose their sons' needless slaughter. Perhaps a mother President could pacify our war-torn planet.

All note America's current inflationary spiral and economic recession, but few proffer plausible explanations or solutions. For many years, labor and managment have short-sightedly profiteered, without concern for quality, durability, or service. Prices and wages have risen unchecked. High pressure tactics have burdened many households with unwanted, superfluous, shoddy "conveniences". Now consumers wax skeptical about purchasing goods and services. Many women successfully and conscientiously manage household budgets; why not corporate or nation budget? Might not our thrifty homemakers minimize waste and right the national economy?

The great ancient civilizations recognized the need for balance in their societies. The Egyptians progressed for thousands of years, enjoying health, justice, emancipation for women and schools for children, and Alexandria, in its zenith under the Ptolemies, had women professors in the University.

All citizens should recognize the capacity of women to govern and share responsibility—to overcome materialism, to foster peace and love, to weed out cruelty, waste and greed.

BUILDING A CLEAN ENVIRONMENT

According to the rules of existence laid out by our Creator, anything that violates Truth is self-destroying. The law of cause and effect keeps the world in balance and enables human beings to exist. Its action is absolutely impartial. The good we do comes back in the form of blessings and the bad returns to plague us. Our present conditions are due to an imbalance in the laws of nature. Violations of the basic principles of existence always bring dire results.

The Incas and the Egyptians, the People of Atlantis, all had as a basic foundation to their religion, the belief that their very lives depended upon pure air, pure water, pure earth and sunshine. It was because they disobeyed these fundamental laws of Nature that the magnificent empires of Egypt, Persia, Greece and Italy succumbed and that the magnificent continent of Atlantis disappeared beneath the waters. They were victimized by soft living, degeneracy and improper food. Mother Nature cannot operate successfully under the present environmental conditions. Our national degradation is a reflection of our ignorance and lack of understanding of our relationship with Nature.

Scientists have never fully understood the totality of God's natural laws. The ecological balance of the natural forces in our land is being rapidly destroyed as man continues to follow his unrealistic notions of his own "superior creative genius." This country was once a fertile land rich with vegetation, a pristine wilderness with beautiful towering forests abounding in wildlife, fast flowing rivers and clear blue lakes, refreshing and teaming with life, a clean air in a bright blue sky that gave vigor and vitality. Freedom comes to the individual from understanding the laws of his own life and conforming to them, thereby subjecting them to his use. Although the workings of both man's technology and nature's systems are complex, many of the problems that have arisen from the collision between them have simple roots. It doesn't require special training to keep a broad perspective and to apply common sense.

Let's keep in mind these few ecological facts: everything comes from somewhere and everything ends up somewhere; all systems and problems are ultimately interrelated; we live on a planet whose resources are infinite. We must hold to a faith in the ability of our own bodies and in the capacity of the earth's ecosystems that Nature has spent millions of years refining and stabilizing, while we try to combine concern for survival with a faith that our individual contributions can make a difference.

Imagine what would happen in our neighborhoods if the fences came down that divide suburban open space into tiny back yards. Something like the recreation of the commons could happen, each family donating some of its sovereign territory to the neighborhood and each receiving more in return. There could be broad open places where children could run and play and communication and new understanding between human beings could blossom.

Every consumer decision we make has an environmental impact. Every time we visit the supermarket, buy a ticket to travel, choose a place to live, our choices have an effect on the quality of the air we breathe and the water we drink, the world we experience with our eyes and ears and nose. Having looked at the market in broad terms, we should be prepared to revise our shopping strategy and as necessary our life style so we can live more ecologically. The environmentally concerned human being should try to minimize consumption while using common sense, the most valuable guide that any consumer can use in making decisions. Ask ourselves these questions: do we need it? If we have it, do we use it? Can we share it? Let's promote recycling in our own home and in our neighborhood.

A modest-sized pine can be bought live in a tub to provide festive decoration indoors for the Christmas Holidays and enjoyment and beauty throughout the year in the front or back yard. Let's learn to walk and ride a bicycle and put the family on bicycles for a day in the country instead of packing them into the car. Noise is a pollutant which we meet at work, in our homes, out of doors and in transit and we have control over many of these pollutants, especially in the home.

The battle for enviromental quality requires that we work through both the individual and institutions, commerce, industry and government. Waiting for the government to "do something" can be like waiting for Godot. We should be interdependent with, not dependent upon, the government. Compare what business leaders say in speeches about pollution with what their companies' advertisments advocate. Let's learn to read the label on the package and buy only what is needed and healthful. Contaminated, unfit foods and cheap surplus "labor-saving" devices will cease to be sold when the market drops because concerned consumers refuse to buy. The ecologically sound way to deal with sewage "waste" disposal is to recognize that sewage is not waste but misplaced fertilizer. There are ecologically sound answers to garbage disposal, such as "digestors" or a worm-powdered refuse disposal project which could replace our incinerators and convert the waste into the finest quality compost for soil enrichment.

Our own bodies, of course, are the most intimate part of our environment, an ecosystem of immense complexity, yet easily cared for by Nature's methods. The commonest cause of disease is primarily overindulgence in the appetites and passions. To combat internal pollution and degeneration of the body, we should eat live, organically grown foods which give vital nourishment to the cells, in amounts and combinations that promote health and well-being, a clean smooth working organism. To combat air pollution in our cities, we should eat little so that the blood stream is able to more easily cleanse and purify our bodies and grow wheatgrass in our homes to purify and freshen the air, absorb carbon dioxide and increase the amount of oxygen available.

In contrast to ancient philosophies which lay great stress on the harmony between human beings and nature, our modern Western culture sharply separates its idea of God from its idea of Nature and looks upon the human race as having a unique place within Creation. In *Our Poisoned Earth and Sky,* Mr. Rodale quotes from an issue of the Royal Bank of Canada's monthly letter: "We need to discard our ideas of 'attacking' the forest, 'bringing under subjugation' the mighty rivers, 'conquering' the mountains, and 'subduing' the prairie. Instead, we need to make the most of nature, as an ally . . ." Go out alone in the woodland in the spring and you will see every leaf, every twig of the trees and plants and vines and shrubs, green in the joy of being, ever grateful to the Creator for giving it life. Sit by a brook or a stream, and in the songs of the brooks and rivers and lakes you will hear them singing the glory of life while ravishing waters dance with Love in water and air. Go out in the purple dusk of sunset and you will find the earth and the mountains and the seas and the sky all bent in audible whispers of prayer that life goes on ever and ever with this omni-present air. Close your eyes and you will find in the heart of your heart the fount spring of this nectar which alone is life.

A Prayer of Praise

Praise be to Thee, O Lord,
For all Thy creatures,
And especially for our Brother, the Sun,
Who gives us the day,
And who shows forth Thy light.
Fair is He and Radiant with great splendor to us,
He is the symbol of Thee, O Lord.

Praise be to Thee, O Lord,
For our sister, the Moon,
And for the Stars.
Thou hast set them clear,
Beautiful and precious in the heaven above.

Praise be to Thee, O Lord,
For our Brother, the Wind,
For the air and the clouds,
For the clear sky and for all weathers,
By which Thou givest life
To all Thy creatures.

Praise be to Thee, O Lord,
For our Brother, Fire,
By whom Thou givest us
Light in the darkness.
He is beautiful and bright,
Courageous and strong.

Praise be to Thee, O Lord,
For our Sister, Water,
Who is useful to us,
Humble, precious and chaste.

Praise be to Thee, O Lord,
For our Mother, the Earth,
Who sustains us and nourishes us,
Bringing forth divers fruits,
Flowers of many colors and the grass.

St. Francis' Canticle to the Sun

FIRST AID

Accidents may be prevented if precautionary steps are taken. Never leave anything on the stairs. See to it that children pick up their toys. Always have a rubber mat in the shower or bathtub. Anticipate trouble, then take the necessary steps to avoid it.

BILIOUSNESS —

This condition is the result of an overtaxed liver and the eating of too much rich food. There is usually a feeling of nausea, upset stomach and feverishness. Food should not be eaten. Take only cool or warm water (room temperature). Vomiting will rid the body of the material that caused the trouble. Biliousness does not last long if you give Nature a chance to correct matters. Lie down in a darkened room and try to relax and go to sleep.

BOILS —

Boils are the result of improper diet. Fresh fruit, sprouts and greens should make up the diet. Apply hot compresses on the boils for several minutes at different times during the day. Keep the compresses hot. In due time, the boils will come to a head and the pus will drain out. Living food will change the nature of the bloodstream, preventing a recurrence of this condition.

BREATHING DIFFICULTY —

If a person is gasping, rub the arms or feet hard, moving toward the heart. I have had many experiences of this nature, and this action never failed me. Blood poisoning sometimes stops circulation; that is why rubbing is so beneficial. If breathing stops completely, mouth-to-mouth resuscitation should be administered immediately and an ambulance should be called. When a person is in the clutches of epilepsy, place person flat on the floor and leave there until they come to.

BROKEN BONES —

Do not get excited. Calmly make the person with broken arm or leg as comfortable as possible until the doctor arrives. It is best not to move them.

CANKERS —

A canker or any other sore in the mouth, on the inside of the cheeks, or on the gums or tongue, is due to too much acidity in the body. This may result from drinking too much coffee, eating too much citrus fruit, or consuming too much candy. Wash out the mouth with fresh chlorophyll juice. Also a little alum on the affected part will help. keeping the mouth open to allow the alum to dry. Drink plenty of water throughout the day to help neutralize the overacid condition of the blood.

COLDS —

Health authorities tell us that crippling colds incapacitate the average person at least one week out of every year. When we feel a cold coming on, either through sniffles or sore throat, the feet should be soaked immediately in very hot water. Of course, it is even better to soak in a hot bath for at least 15 minutes. Then climb into bed, take a hot lemonade, but above all stay away from milk. A heating pad will increase warmth in the body and induce sweating.

Colds, as a rule, can be successfully prevented if the sufferer will stop eating all solid foods and forgo all dairy products. The weakened stomach should be filled with warm lemonade and plenty of water. And an enema should be taken. A cold is merely a health measure whereby the body eliminates toxins and these other steps assist and speed up this elimination. Should the cold persist, the same suggested routine should be followed religiously the following day. There is no reason why anyone with a cold should stop working if rest may be obtained during the night. Going to bed early will help.

Where there is a sore throat, gargle with pure fresh wheatgrass chlorophyll. Wrap the throat with a large towel and allow the throat to sweat out the poisons in the body. Above all, do not worry; know that if you do your part, Nature will do Hers. Scores of families, living Nature's way, do not know what it is to have a cold epidemic in their home, nor do they have to worry about any Asiatic influenza bugs.

CONSTIPATION —

First, eliminate all starches from the diet and substitute fruits, vegetables, sprouts and greens. Take a colonic irrigation if possible to cleanse the colon or take a water enema. Then a half hour later following a water enema, use implants of wheatgrass juice every day for at least three or four weeks until the condition improves. Drinking liquids will also help alleviate constipation.

CUTS —

There are six quarts of blood in the average human body. A cut on a finger is no need for excitement. A person could lose a quart of blood and not pass out. When there is a deep cut, place a flat splint of wood against it and wrap securely, applying pressure to the affected part until the bleeding stops. When there is excessive bleeding from a wound, stop it with a tight band applied between the heart and the wound. A rolled handkerchief or other cloth twisted tightly with a pencil or other object works well. To stop bleeding quickly, soak in chlorophyll for 10 minutes.

FAINTING —

Fainting is caused by overexertion, interrupted digestion and strong emotions. A person who is anemic is more susceptible to fainting than one who is not. If with a person who has fainted, we should bring the body to a sitting position. Standing behind the person, press fingers hard against the temples, then place hands on either side of the neck and rub vigorously downward. Take the lower arms and rub vigorously toward the body. Rub the legs with a squeezing stroke the same way. Cold water on the face is always helpful. As the person regains consciousness, he should be advised to breathe deeply. Fresh air is always very important.

FEVER —

Fevers are the natural build up of heat in the body to kill offending organisms before they can fully take root. In some illnesses, doctors actually induce fever in the patient, for the high temperature burns the toxins in the body. Do not be frightened. Let the sufferer lie down and relax. Cover with a blanket as fevers are often followed by chills. Try to prevent chills; massage the body and place a cold wet facecloth on the forehead. Also, sponge the face and limbs with cold water. Give the patient plenty of cool liquids, preferably a sweet fresh fruit drink—watermelon, orange, and lemon, or apricot. Implants taken before the fever becomes intense will help to detoxify the body and reduce the necessity of the body for fever. If the temperature exceeds 104° F, a physician should be notified.

FOOD POISONING—

Experience shows that virus upsets, allergies, etc., are

nothing more than symptoms of food poisoning. The symptoms are cold, aching bones, bleary eyesight, dizziness, headache, stuffed nose, chills and sleepiness. This condition may cling for a long time if not handled in proper manner and can become serious. Irradiated meat and other contaminated food can bring on this condition. When we feel sickness coming on, we should act at once. If thirsty, drink plenty of water with a little lemon or lime juice added to it. Go to bed, rest and don't worry. Above all, we should not eat anything until we are really hungry. Our digestion may be out of order for several days. If we do eat, we will merely poison our body further as the digestion cannot take care of the food properly. Do not take drugs. Use an enema each morning and if possible a daily one-cup implant of wheatgrass chlorophyll. This implant will give the nourishment we need while we cannot eat.

MINOR HAND BURNS—

Place the hands immediately in cold water. To encourage fast healing, place hand in freshly extracted wheatgrass chlorophyll. This method encourages quick healing and leaves no scars.

HEADACHES —

This testimony speaks for itself: "Dear Dr. Ann, I had been a victim of headaches ever since I was in college more than fifteen years ago. I tried every remedy I ever heard about trying to gain permanent relief. All of them helped a little, but when the newness wore off, the old pain came surging back. After the relief, each new surge seemed worse than the last. I consulted many doctors and paid for countless prescriptions. I had my nerves examined, and I tried chiropractic treatments.

Always the doctors said there was something wrong with my body, but none of them centered upon my stomach. This was done by an elderly woman, a non-doctor, by the way, who told me that all headaches came from an upset stomach. She suggested that I forget cooked foods for a while and follow your uncooked routine for a week to see if I didn't feel better. Naturally, a week did not seem long after all I had suffered, so on November 7, my birthday, I embarked on the good ship 'living food' voyage which I hoped would land me in a paradise of relief. I bought a vegetable grinder and set about preparing my own meals, raising sprouts and greens, etc., and it certainly paid off. I can testify that uncooked food worked miracles as far as headaches were concerned." H.S.M. Missouri.

INSECT BITES —

Most human beings suffer from insect bites inflicted by mosquitoes, gnats, flies, ants. On some persons, these cause redness and swellings around the spot. On others, the effect is merely itching. Rub a little fresh lemon juice on the affected spot, or if wheatgrass chlorophyll is available, bind the spot with a poultice made of wheatgrass pulp.

MENSTRUAL TROUBLES —

There should never be a trace of pain or discomfort during menstrual periods. Of course, tension, unsuitable food, and a host of other things in our modern life help to bring on cramps and headaches that often incapacitate a woman for three or four days. Cut down on the solid food immediately, taking only liquids until comfortable. Apply warm, moist packs to the abdomen. Rest, and above all relax. An enema to cleanse the colon is always in order. Cramps do not just happen. They are the result of incorrect eating habits. A good nutritional pattern will correct the difficulty.

NASAL CONGESTION —

Fill a third of a cup with chlorophyll juice and skim off the top. Place the edge of the cup against upper lip tilting cup slightly, take ten small snuffs. Remove the cup and allow the chlorophyll to run out of nose and throat. The sinuses will hurt a bit as the chlorophyll juice reaches places out of reach of sprays and drops. Where trouble is experienced with any of the nasal passages, the treatment should be done at least three times a day. Instead of merely giving relief, as drugs do, this method eliminates the trouble permanently, assuming proper diet, of course. Therefore, a change of diet is necessary.

Nose Bleed —

This condition seems to be increasing in this country. It is caused by the weakening of the frailest membrane in the body, the interior of the nose. Malnutrition, the lack of sufficient nourishment, is to blame. Sniff up a small amount of freshly squeezed wheatgrass juice into the nostrils. This seems to mend the broken membrane of the interior of the nose. If no wheatgrass juice is available, use cold water and fresh lemon juice.

Skin Troubles —

All skin troubles originate in the stomach and arise from too much heavy food or the eating of improper mixtures of food. Skin conditions are not caused by germs but by tiny organisms festered by an upset digestive tract due to rich foods, etc. The way to eliminate the trouble is through cleanliness and a change of diet.

Skin disorders and eruptions are a warning by Nature that the bloodstream is dangerously filled with poisons. She cannot wait to have these eliminated in the regular way and so sends them directly to the surface of the body in the shape of boils, pimples, etc. These short cuts probably save our lives in many instances since Nature has found it impossible to throw out the dangerous material as rapidly as normal health requires.

(a) Acne —

Acne affects mostly young people from 14 to 20. The cause is a sluggish colon and in most cases constipation. Because the

169

debris in the body, due to slow circulation, cannot be sent through the skin by perspiration, it forms pimples, etc. It is very important to wash the affected skin with wheat blended with water and to rub the area with a rough towel. Chlorophyll juice should then be applied. A person with acne should be careful of sweets, starches and fats.

(b) ECZEMA —

Eczema is not contagious and is a mere eruption of the skin. It is a digestive disturbance occuring in young and old alike. Generally the system is over acid and alkaline foods are necessary. The bowels should be kept open. Use an enema if necessary. The skin should be kept clean with wheat blended with water. Where the eruption itches, it should be bathed with chlorophyll. This tends to prevent scabbing. Eczema is actually a blessing. It is one of Nature's mild warnings that the bloodstream is polluted and that something must be done to clean it.

(c) ITCHING —

The chronic itch is caused by a parasite which lives in the skin and, since it burrows deeply, is hard to dislodge. It is a condition caused by an unhealthy body. A person with a clean bloodstream never has trouble with the skin. Diabetics are generally subject to itchy skin because of the insulin that is taken. Over-acidity will also cause itching. This is remedied by a change in diet. Itching in the female organs is difficult to handle, even by specialists. A change of diet and bathing the affected areas with chlorophyll juice will clear up the problem in a few days.

(d) PSORIASIS —

This health problem is characterized by a rough, reddened, scaly surface of the body. When it appears at the back of the elbows or knees, it shows as small pimples. It sometimes starts this way on the scalp. The best method for relief is to cleanse the colon and change the diet to uncooked foods.

STRAINS AND SPRAINS —

This condition generally causes swelling and is extremely painful. There may be a slight discoloration of the skin because the blood is not circulating properly at that point. In the case of a sprained wrist or ankle, place in hot water and stroke the injured part with your hand toward the head. The stroking sends the blood away from the injured part and allows new healing blood to take its place. This stroking should be continued for some time, perhaps 25 or more minutes, until the part feels comfortable again. This method will reduce the swelling and in cases of light sprains, the swelling will disappear almost at once. However, in the severe situation, the swelling may last for several days.

WARTS —

A wart is an abnormal growth which has been formed because of a disturbance of the cells at a certain spot. Sometimes it is caused by medicines, or it could be the result of other toxins, or faulty diet. The most effective way to eliminate warts is to change the diet to fruit, sprouts, greens and wheatgrass. If it is a protruding wart, encircle it tightly with a silk threat to cut off the blood supply. In a day or so, it will drop off.

BEAUTY THE ORGANIC WAY

True beauty is the radiance of a healthy body, a serene mind and a loving disposition. The external beauty which manifests in our faces and bodies should be the natural, outer radiance of inner beauty. Mother Nature never fails if we cooperate with Her. We need to learn to love and respect the Holy Temple which God has provided us from the dust of the

Earth and give them the proper sustenance they need, physically, mentally and spiritually. A good complexion and radiant beauty depends primarily upon a smooth working body mechanism under the direction of a serene mind. We must be relaxed, get plenty of sleep and have a happy disposition. The nervous system must function normally since worries, tension and other disturbances eventually show up unbecomingly on our faces.

The foundation of all beauty is health. To obtain a glowing skin, clear eyes, a supple, attractive body, we must eat food which gives life and health to our bodies, living, uncooked organic foods. We must watch our digestion carefully, eat sparingly and keep our bodies well nourished and cleansed inside and out. A healthy complexion and soft youthful skin begins with a clean colon and living, uncooked food. Most people do not understand how to use nature to help themselves, how to give their bodies the natural tools to rebuild themselves. When they experience lack of energy, they use crutches such as aspirin, coffee, alcohol and tobacco, which whip the body instead of helping it renew itself.

Many entertainment stars have found the secret of youth. Gloria Swanson, radio, television and movie star, is an example. During her visit to Boston, she confided to me that organically grown foods which contain precious elements have rebuilt her body. She proved how a person could be just as vigorous and lovely at the age of seventy-two as she had been at forty. A natural solution to the problem of health and beauty was discovered by Melvin C. Page, a biochemist in St. Petersburg, Florida. Through his research with thousands of patients who had an imbalance in their body chemistry due to improper diet, he found that their bodies could be rebuilt by vitamins, minerals, and other nutritional elements found only in uncooked food. By following this type of diet, his patients recovered their youth.

The Nobel Prize Foundation, Royal Laplander Academy of Science of Finland, in 1971, awarded me recognition for my work in the field of Youthfulness, commending me for my efforts in regeneration of the human cells and tissues. I want to help people feel young, become their true selves, beautiful, healthy, vibrant and loving persons. I want to share the knowledge of the gifts of nature that have been and will be always available if only we will understand them.

Having myself experienced the fears of age, wrinkled skin, graying hair, overweight, I understand why people desire to be youthful. I can sympathize with that horrible feeling of growing old because at the age of fifty I was an old lady. At that age when most people think about retiring, I decided to change my life style. I began to study Nature to find how I could regain youth. Now twelve years later, the result of my discoveries has brought me to a state of consistent good physical and mental health. My hair has returned to the normal color it was and my weight to the comfortable 119 pounds it had been when I was fifteen years old. Working up to 18 or 20 hours a day, seven days a week, without stopping, I am able to accomplish more mental and physical labor than when I was twenty. But my peak has not yet been reached. I have only begun to realize the value of nature for health and growth.

Artificial aids are not necessary, are expensive and often are harmful to the body. A face uplift to remove sagging muscles, a wig to cover straggly, graying hair, and make up to camouflage failing beauty do not solve the problem. It does no good to cover the skin. The cosmetics now offered to the public are, for the most part, made up of chemicals, of synthetic poisons that harm the skin, only a little in the first application, but through continuous use cause danger and damage to the body. The annual sales of cosmetics has reached its highest mark in history. Reports show that over twelve billion dollars for this form of beauty treatments was expended last year by both men and women.

Most people have jars of unused and partially used creams on their shelves. They do not do what those people thought they would do and there is a valid reason for this. These cosmetics are full of harsh chemicals so they either irritated, were too greasy, too dry, etc. As a result of this tremendous use of these so-called "beauty improvement devices", doctors report that human ailments are increasing at an alarming rate. Skin problems and ill health are manifested through cracked lips, discolored fingernails, and other distressing conditions which send the sufferers to specialists of one kind or another.

An explanation about skin will reveal why it is necessary to wash often and have healthy food. The skin has two main layers: the inner layer called the "dermis", which serves as a matrix, and the outer layer called the "epidermis" which serves as a defense layer against bacteria, which would otherwise invade the skin. The inner layer serves as an eliminative organ and body temperature regulator. It contains nerve endings and sweat glands which rid the body of waste material and water. This layer also has oil glands which lubricate the skin and emit electricity which gives life and radiance to the skin. In order for the skin the be radiant, the glands and blood vessels must have living nourishment. The outer layer constantly sheds, replacing itself with new skin. The dead skin and waste particles and moisture must be removed by daily washing with a good, natural soap and water to prevent dry and wrinkled skin.

Hair should be washed with a natural soap or shampoo which contains no chemicals. Lemon is a purifier to the hair as well as to the scalp and is an ideal rinse. Squeeze the juice of two or three lemons into a bowl, adding four times as much water as juice. Soap the hair well, then rinse thoroughly, and rinse again with lemon juice. Be sure to have your rinse ready. Dandruff due to faulty diet may be corrected speedily through the eating of uncooked organic food and thoroughly brushing of the hair daily with a wire wig brush. For relief, rub coconut oil into scalp and cover the head with a steaming, wet bath towel, leaving it there for a full fifteen minutes.

Before we retire at night, we should wash our face thoroughly and rinse it well, using a natural sponge—sometimes called a cucumber sponge—which is much better than a face cloth and equally good for the whole body. A beauty pack should be applied to the face once or twice a week. This will help to keep blemishes and pimples from the face. Two wonderful packs are the yolk of an egg applied over the face and left there until it dries, and honey that is unheated. This type of pack could well be left on all night; that is, if we sleep alone. If the skin is oily, lemon is a great aid.

For dry skin, a pack of mashed ripe banana mixed with sunflower oil is excellent. While the beauty pack is doing its work, let's relax, listen to music or meditate. After fifteen minutes, remove the pack, washing face carefully. For very dry skin, a little vegetable or olive oil after the pack is good; a ripe avocado is excellent as it is a natural type of cream which eliminates dryness and nourishes at the same time. Massaging the face gently in an upward motion especially around the mouth, softens the expression and brings a foundation of stronger muscles under the skin, lessening the tendency toward wrinkles and set, stern lines. However, care should be taken not to apply too much pressure in the region of the eyes since the underlying muscles in these areas are comparatively weak and easily injured. For oily skin, we should use lemon juice instead or rub freshly cup-up potato over the face.

The sins committed on our bodies manifest in the face as lines and sagging tissues. Have face wrinkles vanish in a second. Gather a finger full of hair above the ears on each side of the head and tie the two strands on top of the head, pulling the hair very tight. We may cover the place with a band or wig to match the hair. This only removes wrinkles as long as the hair remains tightly pulled, of course. Naturally we are working to remove these wrinkles permanently. Whistling is the best type of exercise and is a tissue builder. Making faces, as children call it, is splendid, but do not do this in front of anyone! A calm, easy disposition will prevent wrinkles on the forehead. A good exercise for the face is to open the mouth wide and stick out the tongue. This helps to increase the circulation in the face and aids in eliminating any toxic deposits that might be present.

The eyes are the most attractive feature of the face. They are the "windows of the soul". Tired eyes have ruined the appearance of more people than wrinkles, falling hair or sallow skin. Tired eyes cannot be erased by cosmetics. They should be bathed with an eye cup filled with fresh chloropyll twice a day.

One very good method to aid beauty, besides improving general health, is to take ice water or ice cubes and leave on the face for a very short period of time. This method is good to apply early in the morning when we first get up. It tightens the skin and at the same time really wakes us up. Have you often wondered how the Swedish girls keep their lovely skin so radiant? I will share their secret. They take a medium bristle brush and brush their entire body to wake it up each morning and bring the blood to the surface so it can carry off inner impurities. An air bath as long as time permits upon arising is very beneficial. Benjamin Franklin learned this secret in France in those days when air baths were common in Europe.

A pleasing supple figure is easily achieved and maintained through healthful living. This does not mean skinny or undernourished; a healthy body is not underweight any more than it is overweight. A nourishing diet of living foods and plenty of exercise will give us good health and the "perfect-figure" we talk about so wistfully. Flabby arms, a sagging stomach and weak back are one of the results of our many labor-saving devices in the home. Pushups are wonderful to tone the muscles in these areas. No special time or place is needed. Whether we are preparing dinner, making the beds or watching a television show, whenever we happen to think of it, we should take a moment to do a pushup or two. Lie on the stomach with hands placed flat on the floor under the shoulders, feet resting on the bottoms (balls) of the turned up toes. Slowly straighten arms, lifting the entire body from the toes off the floor, keeping back straight, maintain horizontal position for a moment and then slowly come straight down. This will firm up those flabby arm muscles and greatly strengthen the back.

Common sense tells us that good care of the feet is of vital importance to health. My heart sickens when I see how women throw their feet entirely out of natural lines through the wearing of high heels. Experience has demonstrated to me that nothing can bring on old age quicker than neglected or abused feet. Overweight, high heels, cramping shoes and improper diet cause ulcers, varicose veins, running sores, etc. These outbreaks are the only method through which Mother Nature can obtain relief from intolerable conditions within the body. Experience has shown that the best method of meeting all foot conditions, chronic or acute, is a basin of water, as hot as we can stand it, in which the water rises only to the ankles. Fifteen minutes a day for aching feet will afford the body more relaxation and relief than a full day at the beach. Following the foot bath, dry feet well, oil them thoroughly and be ready for spot therapy to relieve upset conditions in any part of the body. Two persons, working together on each other's feet, can accomplish wonders. With the thumb, press the desired spot hard and move the thumb slowly in a small circle.

ESPECIALLY FOR OUR PETS

Albert Schweitzer composed this prayer, "Dear God, protect and bless all creatures that have breath; save them from all evil and let them live in peace and quietness."

A pet is a good example. A pet is a live animal; it has feelings, it desires love and attention. Pets are like children and must be provided with the necessities of a good life, housing, proper diet, discipline, exercise, sunlight and fresh air, and a comfortable place to sleep. They should be encouraged to eat everything uncooked and should have at least two regular meals a day to prevent overeating. Snackitis is just as harmful for our pets as for ourselves. It is more important for pets to be underweight than overweight. If a pet refuses to eat, it is a sign that he or she is not well and Nature has curbed its appetite. Do not worry or encourage the little animal to eat; just make sure there is plenty of fresh water, with a bundle of wheatgrass in it, available. The pet may gulp the wheatgrass, as a medicine, and then throw up the poisons from the stomach. As with humans, a pet should never have drugs, injections or vitamins in pill form, as these pollute the bloodstream and cause serious side-effects. A pet should definitely have a natural elimination of waste material every day. A bird should have plenty of gentle sunlight and not be kept cooped up all day in a small cage where its wings cannot be properly exercised. All domestic animals need some sunshine and exercise each day.

I consider Precious, my little woolly monkey, one of the most wonderful pets anyone could love. What a splendid disposition; she spreads joy to whomever she meets. She's a baby who never grows up. The old expression of "monkey see, monkey do" applies absolutely to Precious. She watches every move I make and seeks to imitate my actions. When I am changing dresses, she watches closely and tries to discard her own dress. If I offer her some new food, she refuses even to taste it until I take a bite of it. Then she hastily follows suit.

Puzzled veterinarians ask me, "Why has pet blindness increased at an alarming rate?" I answer the obvious—deficient and chemicalized food. Here is a simple tasty meal which will benefit dogs, cats and any other domesticated animals. Grind or finely chop one cup of slightly sprouted wheat and one cup of mung bean sprouts. Add one handful of cut-up wheatgrass and one-half cup of fish or meat, whatever the pet enjoys. Add ground carrots if he likes them. Avoid canned food of any kind. We should ease our pets into this diet until they become accustomed to the new food. Wheat or sunflower milk is wonderful for a meal. Living, uncooked foods will keep our pets in "romping good health" and loving disposition.

The most enjoyable meal Precious has is breakfast of wheat "milk". While I am preparing her breakfast, Precious usually sits patiently in a chair and eagerly watches everything I do. She drinks out of the side of the cup just like any human being. She just loves her wheat "milk", and also coconut water, which keeps her bowels in order. If a pet is sluggish in any way, coconut water will often solve the problem. Precious is also extremely fond of fruit at lunch and all the sprouts and grated vegetables and special sauces which we make here for our guests for the evening meal. I always feed parakeets seed twice a week, see that they get green leafy vegetables and ripe pieces of pear, apple or other mild fruit, and keep a spray of wheatgrass in their water. My pet raccoon and skunk live together and feed together on the same live food. I place two dishes of food for them—one of fruit and one of vegetables. These little animals wisely, instinctively, eat only one dish at a time, or even one kind in a day. The raccoon seems to prefer vegetables, the skunk fruit, and seed for extra protein. As time goes on, we find that the directions for the care of the pet come from within, just like caring for the human family.

I breathe a constant prayer of thanks that I have eaten no animal product for many years. One of the most beloved peacemakers of our times, Mahatma Ghandi, who was a vegetarian, said, "It ill becomes us to invoke in our daily prayers the blessings of God, the Compassionate, if we in turn will not practice elementary compassion towards our fellow creatures." A human being is ethical only when life, as such, is sacred to them, that of plants and animals as that of their fellow humans, and when they devote themselves helpfully to all life that is in need of help. The ethic of the relation of human beings to one another is not something apart by itself; it is only a particular relation which results from and within the universal one.

This reverence for life was taught by all the Great Teachers. Jesus, Krishna and Gotama the Buddha were pictured as Good Shepherds. Jesus said that we "must respect the brotherhood of life. Whoever is not kind to every form of life—to man, to beast, to bird and all creeping things—cannot expect the blessings of the Holy One." Gotama the Buddha became known as the Lord of Compassion for his teachings of kindness and helpfulness towards all living things. The Hindu Scriptures tell us that "wise people see the same Divine Breath in the Absolute, in worms, insects, in the outcasts, in the dog, in the elephant, in beasts, in cattle, in gadflies and gnats." (Bhagavad Gita)

Jewish religion teaches that "to cause the slightest pain in any living animal, however low it may be in the scale of creation, is a sin which is worth many laws to prevent." In spite of this, the Jews are carrying on with their cruel method of "Kosher" slaughtering. Mohammed said that "there are no beasts on the earth nor birds which fly with their wings which do not belong, like yourself, to God's family." Yet even in our times Moslems sacrifice lambs, goats, and even camels. This act is breaking the law of nature. Man's "dominion" over the animals has seen an unending massacre. In one single year, the number of animals slaughtered for food, or otherwise unnecessarily exploited, injured, maimed, tortured and killed by vivisection, "experiments", trapping, hunting, etc., is over 15,000 million. No wonder we have wars!

The growing child naturally loves little God-guided creatures and is given pets and cuddly animal toys in order to nurture that loving and protective instinct. Many children feel toward an animal smaller than themselves and dependent upon their care greater tenderness than they feel toward human beings. How great must be their confusion and pain, then, when in school they are taught that their normal respect for life is just "squeamishness" to be overcome and their emotional attachments to living creatures is suppressed. In the name of "science", thousands of American youngsters are being encouraged, even paid, to torture and kill harmless animals. They practice "surgical" disection on live animals, mice are often starved to death to test the effects of vitamins and vitamin deficiencies, small animals are made to spin in dryers until they paralyze themselves to death. In one high school in Buffalo, they are taught to blow pepper, dust and smoke into the lungs of mice to provoke "violent shutting off of the glottis", toxicity tests to find out what doses of nicotine will kill animals, substitution of external artificial hearts.

Skin transplants, amputations of organs and poison injections are going on every day, as well as routine and periodic transfer of cancer cells to healthy animals. "It is nothing short of butchery", says an SPCA official. Agricultural research stations experimentally infect steers with any number of devastating diseases and coldly study the animal while it suffers and dies. At the New England Regional Primate Research Center, owl monkeys are injected with a virus to produce a form of leukemia. So what is the Primate Center going to do about curing this "uncurable disease" in these little sufferers? Very often the animal's death is very slow and painful.

It is very strange that although this type of animal torture has gone on for many centuries, not one single thing to aid human beings, well or ill, has ever emerged from such cruelty. In fact, the health and well-being of humans continues to decline rapidly, our life span grows shorter. If this strikes you in the same manner it has me, sit right down and write a letter to your U.S. Senator or Representative and tell him in unmistakable words that even he can understand that your vote will go elsewhere in the next election unless he bestirs himself and does something constructive to end this horrible system which for centuries has disgraced humanity. For this end, we must tell our elected officials that no matter how many millions of dollars may be spent on such research, seeking cures, the effort is wasted. The human body has to do the healing, and without proper nourishment the body cannot heal itself.

There is something about the unfailing affection of God-guided creatures which seemingly cannot be equalled through the use of the free will by human beings. As a young herdsgirl, in war torn Europe, I saw this loving attribute demonstrated by a nondescript mongrel left in the care of a relative who lived nearby. The disgraceful episode began before I was born. The little boy who had been the constant companion of Spotty for over six years departed with his parents for America and the animal was left in the care of his aunt. The dog, tied to the stump in front of the house in the dusk of the evening, had watched his master disappear down the road in the wagon. Its plaintiff wails that night earned for it a severe beating by its none-too-gentle new protector.

I must have been at least seven years old when grandmother called the plight of Spotty to my attention. During the day the dog roamed the village but every evening as darkness fell it took its position by the stump in the yard. There it stood immovable looking wistfully down the road where the wagon had vanished. Summer, spring, fall and winter, no matter what the weather, it would take that place at dusk and sitting by the stump yearningly watch the distant road. Often I used to join it there, wondering why its master did not at least write to his aunt about the little animal. But no letter ever came—yet little Spotty did not forget.

The lone vigil ended when I was nine years old, one chilly night in March. The afternoon snow had turned to a freezing rain. Grandmother, attending a sick woman, was returning home at dusk and found a shivering Spotty crouching by the stump, its brown eyes upon the distant road. Grandmother, her big heart touched, gathered the shaking little animal in her great cloak and brought it home. Together we fed it warm goat milk and that night it slept beside Star on my feet in the bunk. But next morning it was dead. Its long vigil had been unrewarding—its master seemingly had forgotten.

Grandmother buried the tiny creature near our woodpile. As she patted home the last shovel of dirt, she turned to me and said in a low voice; "Never forget Spotty, Annetta. This tiny God-guided creature was much closer to the Almighty than its master who, under the wonders of the new world, forgot the faithful friend he had kissed goodbye. Only human beings, with their distorted free wills, forget. God-guided creatures never do. Jesus said, 'Come to me, as a little child.' I would paraphrase, 'Come to me, unspoiled as a little soul of the fields or forests.' "

ABOUT DR. ANN WIGMORE

As the founder of Hippocrates Health Institute, Dr. Ann Wigmore has dedicated her life to teaching others the value of living food. Born in Lithuania in 1909, she was raised by her grandmother, who gave her unwaivering confidence in the immense healing power of nature. Dr. Wigmore spent years experimenting to find simple, healthy, and inexpensive ways to grow food indoors, such as the now popular technique of sprouting. Much of her philosophy is as old as Hippocrates himself who taught that if given the correct nourishment, the body will heal itself, and advised, *Let food be your medicine.*

In 1963, under her direction, the Hippocrates Health Institute became a philanthropic, non-sectarian, non-profit organization and study center implementing the principles of living food, wheatgrass chlorophyll, and care of the body for the restoration of vibrant health. Countless are those who have studied and healed themselves there, or who have profited from the knowledge of others who returned eager to teach and help.

In a desire to share her knowledge as broadly as possible, Dr. Wigmore has authored over fifteen books, distributing over one million copies. She has lectured in twenty countries. Her ongoing healing work, with decades of experience backing it, has given others a greater understanding and appreciation of the healer within.

WHAT IS THE HIPPOCRATES PROGRAM?

We offer a two-week program* in which the guests are provided a cleansing and nourishing diet prepared from un-cooked foods and sprouted seeds, grains, fermented foods and juices. Chlorophyll-rich greens are eaten as salads and used in juice form. Daily enemas hasten the cleansing process which helps to restore the body to health.

There are daily classes in physiology, sprouting, and food preparation, and instruction on how to grow food in one's own kitchen. Guests also do their own planting and sprouting and make fermented foods and drinks. A daily exercise program teaches the importance of flexibility, proper posture, and deep breathing and spiritual unfoldment.

WHY LEARN BY DOING?—

Learning by doing is the quickest way to learn and the best way to remember and help to build a healthy lifestyle. Learning by doing will prepare one to carry on the program successfully at home, and continue to improve the total health.

WHAT YOU CAN DO TO PREPARE FOR YOUR VISIT—

Preparation is not essential, but it would be helpful to read *Be Your Own Doctor*. My successful work in the health field for over 30 years assures me that the body does not fail to heal itself when given a chance.

If one wishes to obtain maximum benefits, one can get an early start at home. Before you come, increase your intake of fresh vegetables, greens, sprouts, fruits and their juices.

FINANCIAL ARRANGEMENTS—

Bank checks, cash, or major credit cards are acceptable for tuition, literature, and health equipment.

*(Longer or shorter stays may be arranged if necessary.)

HOW TO RESERVE A SPACE IN OUR COURSE—

Give us a phone call or write to learn the earliest availability. The number is 1-617-267-9525.

HIPPOCRATES HEALTH INSTITUTE PROFESSIONAL INTENSIVE PROGRAM—

Two weeks of learning Nature's simple laws in a way that will enable you to bring a new dimension to the work that you do. As a professional, you already know the rewards of helping people to help themselves. With this program, you can help them to experience increased health, vitality and better concentration. Call for arrangements, even if you can stay only one week.

Our program emphasizes a live-foods program, exercise classes and positive thinking techniques. By learning to grow much of your own organic, life-giving food, you can help reduce the runaway cost of eating. In addition, you will enjoy being able to "Learn by Doing" in the company of others who are also pioneering new alternatives, a way for survival.

Come to "The Mansion" and see what Hippocrates can offer you. The Professional Intensive Program can be taken during any two weeks.

HIPPOCRATES HEALTH MINISTRY PROGRAM—

The Hippocrates Health Ministry Program, a ten-week intensive training program based on Dr. Wigmore's living food nutrition work of the past 30 years, is held three times a year, beginning in the months of January, May, and September. The ministry program consists of a balanced work-study experience of classroom study and "Learn by Doing." The classes are designed to teach and expose the student to various subjects in the field of holistic health. These subjects include: health and diet, anatomy, physiology, counseling, public speaking, iridology, massage, bio-energetics, positive thinking, and many more. To gain the experience of running a health center, the student also assists in the different departments at the Institute. These departments include: office, kitchen, public relations, farmwork, planting, and exercise.

The Health Ministry Program is essentially a learning program set up for dedicated, responsible individuals who wish to learn and then teach the Living Food Program to others. The graduated Health Ministers often visit different communities, schools, homes, and attend seminars, workshops, and conventions where they introduce the Living Food Program to others.

Applications must be reviewed a month prior to the opening date, to insure acceptance. If you are interested, please contact the Hippocrates Health Institute for more information concerning this wonderful program. We are at 25 Exeter Street, Boston, Massachusetts, 02116. Phone 617-267-9525.

For a current list of books and prices in the Hippocrates Health Series and a list of live food equipment and health aids, available at a low cost, write to:

Hippocrates Health Institute
25 Exeter Street
Boston, MA 02116
(617) 267-9525